FF 15

Human Papillomaviruses and Cervical Cancer

Human Papillomaviruses and Cervical Cancer
Biology and Immunology

Edited by

PETER L. STERN

Paterson Institute for Cancer Research,
Christie CRC Research Centre, Manchester

and

MARGARET A. STANLEY

Department of Pathology, University of Cambridge

OXFORD UNIVERSITY PRESS
OXFORD   NEW YORK   TOKYO
1994

Oxford University Press, Walton Street, Oxford OX2 6DP
Oxford New York Toronto
Delhi Bombay Calcutta Madras Karachi
Kuala Lumpur Singapore Hong Kong Tokyo
Nairobi Dar es Salaam Cape Town
Melbourne Auckland Madrid
and associated companies in
Berlin Ibadan

Oxford is a trade mark of Oxford University Press

Published in the United States
by Oxford University Press Inc., New York

A catalogue record for this book is available from the British Library

Library of Congress Cataloging in Publication Data
Human papillomaviruses and cervical cancer : biology and immunology /
edited by Peter L. Stern and Margaret A. Stanley.
Includes bibliographical references and index.
1. Cervix uteri—Cancer—Etiology. 2. Papillomavirus diseases.
3. Cervix uteri—Cancer—Pathophysiology. I. Stern, Peter L. II. Stanley, Margaret A.
[DNLM: 1. Cervix Neoplasms—etiology. 2. Papillomavirus—pathogenicity.
3. Cervix Neoplasms—immunology. 4. Papillomavirus—immunology. WP 480 H9183 1994]
RC280.U8H863 1994 616.99'466—dc20 93—47419

ISBN 0 19 854796 X

Typeset by Apex Products, Singapore
Printed in Great Britain on acid-free paper by St. Edmundsbury Press,
Bury St Edmunds, Suffolk

Preface

Cervical cancer is a major disease worldwide with 500 000 new cases diagnosed each year. Through epidemiological studies, an association has been established with human papillomavirus (HPV) infection throughout the pathological spectrum of this disease. Studies of the molecular and biological basis for the role of HPV in cervical lesions involves clinicians, virologists, cell and molecular biologists, and most recently immunologists. This book is a timely review of HPV infection in cervical cancer and provides a background to the potential for immunological intervention. We are on the threshold of attempts to implement and evaluate such approaches, and this volume seeks to discuss the relevant issues but also deals with the fundamentals of HPV and the spectrum of cervical disease.

Hilary Buckley defines the problem from the clinicopathological standpoint (Chapter 1) while John Arrand outlines the basic molecular genetics of human papillomaviruses (Chapter 2). Jan Walboomers and colleagues then evaluate methods for detecting the latter in cervical lesions (Chapter 3) and the implications of this in epidemiological terms are critically discussed by Ciaran Woodman (Chapter 4). The functions of viral products are discussed in relation to oncoproteins in cancer by Karen Vousden (Chapter 5), and in the natural history of infection in cervical epithelium by Margaret Stanley (Chapter 6). The next chapters deal with the measurement of immunity to HPV and the prospects for immunological intervention in cervical disease. Detection of serological responses to HPV proteins and potential in diagnosis is addressed by Lutz Gissmann and Martin Muller (Chapter 7). The search for cell-mediated immunity to HPV and the prospects for vaccine design are discussed in Chapter 8 by Hans Stauss and Peter Beverley. The implications of modulation of expression of the major histocompatibility products in cervical neoplasia are reviewed in Chapter 9 by Peter Stern and Margaret Duggan-Keen. The final three chapters concentrate on prospects for immunological intervention: Saveria Campo dealing with animal model systems (Chapter 10); Huw Davies reviewing immunological aspects of cutaneous warts, and finally the editors take the liberty of a critical evaluation of the 'real politik' for human vaccination programmes.

Individual chapters have been written so that the reader, irrespective of level or discipline, can follow the text and each is integrated so that the book as a whole provides insight into the most relevant scientific issues of HPV and cervical cancer. This book will provide an interface for students, scientists, and clinicians with a realistic and critical evaluation of the advances and problems in the implementation of immunologically based prophylactic and therapeutic strategies in HPV associated disease.

We thank all our colleagues for their various contributions but particularly Elaine Mercer for her expert help in the preparation of this manuscript. Finally the editors and all the authors are indebted to the European Concerted Action 'Immunology of Human Papillomavirus and Vaccine Development', which has been critical in the development of the scientific interactions that made this volume possible.

Manchester and Cambridge   P. L. S.
March 1994   M. A. S.

Contents

3   Detection of genital human papillomavirus infections: Critical review of methods and prevalence studies in relation to cervical cancer   41
JAN M. M. WALBOOMERS *et al.*

6   Virus–keratinocyte interactions in the infectious cycle 116
Margaret A. Stanley

Contributors

John R. Arrand, Department of Molecular Biology, Cancer Research Campaign Laboratories, Paterson Institute for Cancer Research, Christie CRC Research Centre, Manchester M20 9BX, England

Peter C. L. Beverley, Imperial Cancer Research Fund Tumour Immunology Unit, University College London Medical School, 91 Riding House Street, London W1P 8BT, England

C. Hilary Buckley, Department of Reproductive Pathology, St Mary's Hospital, Whitworth Park, Manchester M13 0JH, England

M. Saveria Campo, The Beatson Institute for Cancer Research, Cancer Research Campaign Laboratories, Garscube Estate, Bearsden, Glasgow G61 1BD, Scotland

Huw Davies, Division of Life Sciences, Infection and Immunity Research Group, Kings College, Camden Hill Road, London, W8 7AH, England

Margaret Duggan-Keen, Department of Immunology, Cancer Research Campaign Laboratories, Paterson Institute for Cancer Research, Christie CRC Research Centre, Manchester M20 9BX, England

Lutz Gissman, Forschungsschwerpunkt Angewandte Tumorvirologie Deutsches Krebsforschungszentrum, Heidelberg, Germany

Martin Muller, Forschungsschwerpunkt Angewandte Turmorvirologie Deutsches Krebsforschungszentrum, Heidelberg, Germany

Margaret A. Stanley, Department of Pathology, University of Cambridge, Division of Virology, Tennis Court Road, Cambridge CB2 1QP, England

Hans J. Stauss, Imperial Cancer Research Fund Tumour Immunology Unit, University College London Medical School, 91 Riding House Street, London W1P 8BT, England

Peter L. Stern, Department of Immunology, Cancer Research Campaign Laboratories, Paterson Institute for Cancer Research, Christie CRC Research Centre, Manchester M20 9BX, England

Karen H. Vousden, Ludwig Institute for Cancer Research, St Mary's Hospital Medical School, Norfolk Place, London W2 1PG, England

Jan M. M. Walboomers, Ana-Maria de Roda Husman, Adrian J. C. van den Brule, Peter J. F. Snijders and Chris J. L. M. Meijer, Department of Pathology, University Hospital Amsterdam, The Netherlands

Ciaran Woodman, Centre for Cancer Epidemiology, Christie Hospital NHS Trust, Manchester M20 9BX, England

1 The pathology of cervical intra-epithelial neoplasia, carcinoma and human papillomavirus infection

C. HILARY BUCKLEY

1.1 Introduction

The uterine cervix is one of the tissues forming the lower female genital tract, a term which also encompasses the vagina and vulva. Whilst this text is concerned with the cervix uteri, it must be remembered that human papillomavirus (HPV) infection, intra-epithelial neoplasia, and carcinoma may affect all these tissues simultaneously or asynchronously. Disease in the cervix, therefore, often forms part of a field change in the lower genital tract, and this may influence the course of the patient's disease and modify their clinical management.

HPV infection and intra-epithelial neoplasia in the cervix is most commonly suspected following a cervical smear, and is usually confirmed by a directed biopsy of the cervix taken during a colposcopic examination. The nature of these specimens, the limitations of these techniques, and the morphology of the lesions is discussed below.

The physiological changes and pathological processes encountered in the cervix are closely related and a knowledge of both is essential to an understanding of the morphological manifestations of HPV infection and cervical neoplasia.

1.2 The normal cervix

The normal cervix is covered on its outer, or lower, surface by a non-keratinizing, stratified squamous epithelium which is continuous below with the squamous epithelium lining the vagina, and above with the mucus-secreting columnar epithelium lining the endocervical canal and crypts (Fig. 1.1). The junction between the two epithelia normally coincides with the external cervical os but this is not a constant relationship. At puberty, during pregnancy (particularly the first one), and in some steroid contraceptive

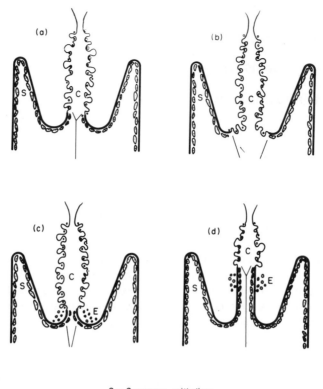

S = Squamous epithelium
C = Columnar epithelium
E = Endocervical glands deep to
    metaplastic squamous epithelium

Fig. 1.1 A diagrammatical representation of the position of the squamocolumnar junction at different ages, and the distribution of the squamous and columnar epithelium on the cervix: (a) 'original' squamocolumnar junction; (b) endocervical eversion (ectropion) with 'original' squamocolumnar junction; (c) transformation zone with 'new' squamocolumnar junction; (d) squamocolumnar junction within endocervical canal after menopause. Reproduced by kind permission from Coleman and Evans (1988).

users, changes in the shape and volume of the cervix result in the squamo-columnar junction being carried out onto the anatomical ectocervix, thus exposing the tissues previously found in the lower endocervical canal, to the vagina. This latter area forms a so-called cervical ectopy or, less appropriately, an ectropion. An understanding of the processes occurring in a cervical ectopy, which is a physiological process, are essential to an understanding of neoplastic processes in the cervix because it is in the area of the cervical ectopy that the majority of intra-epithelial and invasive neoplasms of the cervix develop.

The surface of an ectopy has a villous structure, each villus having a central core of delicate connective tissue supplied by a central capillary, and covered by columnar epithelium.

Under physiological conditions, the columnar epithelium of the ectopy undergoes squamous metaplasia, thus restoring the squamocolumnar junction to the external os. Metaplasia is detected first at the periphery of the ectopy, and is signalled by the appearance of so-called reserve cells beneath the columnar epithelium (Fig. 1.2). These cells gradually become stratified beneath the layer of columnar cells, and assume the morphological features of squamous epithelium (Fig. 1.3). Finally, the columnar cells are lost, and a mature stratified squamous epithelium, in which the vascular pattern of the ectopy is preserved, replaces the columnar epithelium. This epithelium is often less well glycogenated than the original squamous epithelium and a sharp line of demarcation marks the boundary between the original and the metaplastic epithelium. The area of metaplastic squamous epithelium forms what is described as the transformation zone. In younger women, particularly those under the age of 35 years, the metaplastic squamous epithelium of the transformation zone lies on the anatomical ectocervix and is accessible to examination and inspection. In women over the age

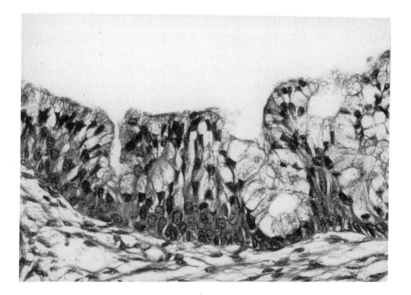

Fig. 1.2 Reserve cell hyperplasia. The epithelium is stratified: the surface layer is composed of mucus-secreting columnar epithelium and the reserve cells, which are small and more darkly staining, form the basal layers.

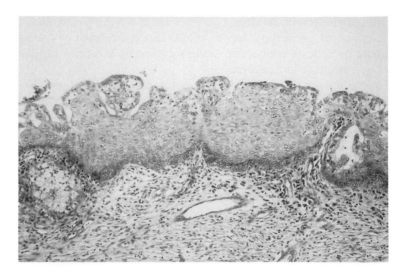

Fig. 1.3 Immature metaplastic squamous epithelium covers the surface of the transformation zone. Endocervical crypts, which are lined by a columnar epithelium, can be seen beneath the stratified squamous epithelium.

of 30 and, to an increasing degree in those over the age of 35 years, the transformation zone is withdrawn into the endocervical canal and thus comes to lie beyond the directly visible range of the examining clinician (Fig. 1.1).

The surface of the endocervical canal, and hence the tissues of the ectopy, form a complex series of invaginations or crypts, and during the formation of the transformation zone the squamous metaplastic process often extends into the underlying crypts which are up to 0.7 cm deep.

1.3 Morphological evidence of HPV infection in the lower genital tract

HPV infection has been implicated in the development of condylomata, intra-epithelial neoplasia, and invasive tumours of the cervix. It is often believed that neoplastic processes associated with HPV are limited to squamous epithelium but evidence is accumulating that HPV may also be important in the development of columnar cell lesions.

The commonest morphological manifestation of HPV infection in the lower genital tract is the *condyloma acuminatum* or genital wart. These are usually the result of infection by HPV types 6 and 11, and are exophytic,

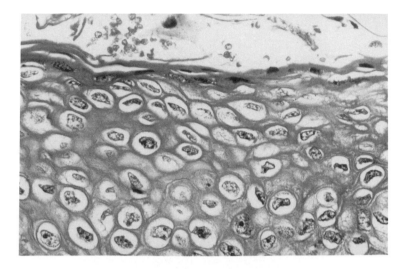

Fig. 1.4 Koilocytes: the nuclei are enlarged, hyperchromatic and have a wrinkled, irregular outline. There is a cavity in the surrounding cytoplasm which has a clearly defined margin.

papillary lesions composed of short or long fronds of connective tissue covered by an acanthotic squamous epithelium. They are often multiple.

In the cervix and vagina, the epithelium covering the condyloma is usually parakeratotic whilst in the vulva it is more commonly hyperkeratotic. This reflects the type of epithelium normally occuring in these sites. Characteristic cellular changes in the epithelium include individual cell keratinization, multinucleation, and koilocytotic atypia (KA) (Fig. 1.4). The latter is regarded as the hallmark of HPV infection. The cells are characterized by the presence of perinuclear cytoplasmic vacuolation, and nuclear enlargement, hyperchromasia, and irregularity. HPV can be identified in such cells, but not constantly, and the proportion of HPV-containing koilocytes varies according to the method chosen to detect the virus.

HPV infection does not always result in the formation of the typical papillary lesion. It may also lead to the development of non-condylomatous wart virus infection or so-called flat condylomata (Fig. 1.5). These are not visible to the naked eye, and the cellular changes are usually detected only in a cervical smear or biopsy, and their site identified at colposcopy. The flat condyloma, or wart, is characterized by the same range of epithelial cytological changes as the *condyloma acuminatum* but the lesion is not raised above the adjacent surface. The epithelium is frequently (though not invariably) parakeratotic or, less commonly, hyperkeratotic and the stratum corneum may, occasionally, form a series of peaks or spikes, an

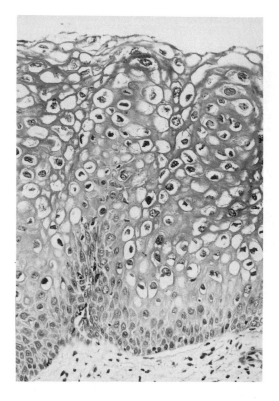

Fig. 1.5 A flat condyloma, or non-condylomatous wart virus infection, of the cervix. The cells in the basal layers are of normal appearance but there are koilocytes in the upper layers.

appearance described as a spiky condyloma (Fig. 1.6). A cervical smear, in which only the surface cells of the epithelium are sampled may, therefore, in such cases fail to reveal the diagnostic koilocytes. In the immature metaplastic squamous epithelium of the transformation zone, the virus may also lead to the development of small filiform papillae covered by immature metaplastic squamous epithelium in which koilocytes are infrequently seen.

It should be emphasized that the presence of KA in a cervical smear does not necessarily mean that the lesion is on the cervix. A cervical smear may also contain cells shed from a lesion on the vaginal vault, and even in those women with an identifiable cervical wart there are often also flat or papillary condylomata in the vaginal vault. The appearance of the condylomatous lesions in the various sites may differ. Some may have all the typical features whilst others may simply be foci of poorly glycogenated

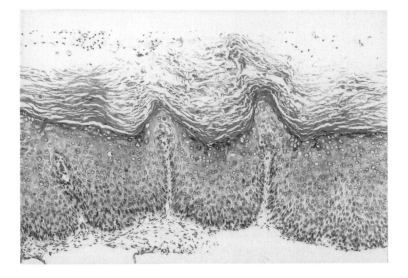

Fig. 1.6 A spiky condylomatous lesion which is covered by a thick layer of keratin, most of which is anucleate. Smears from these lesions may fail to reveal any diagnostic features.

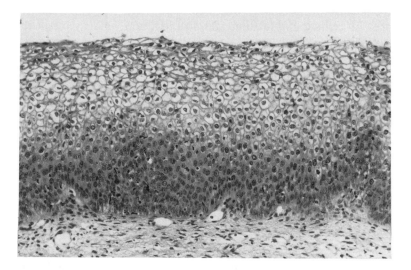

Fig. 1.7 A flat condyloma with basal cell hyperplasia. There is replication of the basal layers of the epithelium but the cells are regular in shape and size. The normality of the cells distinguishes the condition from intra-epithelial neoplasia.

squamous epithelium with occasional KA, and parakeratosis. The virus which is identified within the constituent cells of these various lesions may be of a different type or the same type as the virus present in the cervical lesion.

In some flat condylomata there may be replication of the epithelial basal layers, so-called basal cell hyperplasia. This appearance can be distinguished from intra-epithelial neoplasia by the absence of cytological atypia (Fig. 1.7).

1.4   HPV infection and cervical intra-epithelial neoplasia

HPV infection may result not only in the development of condylomatous lesions but may also be associated with intra-epithelial neoplasia in the same or adjacent epithelium. The intra-epithelial neoplasm may affect either the squamous, or columnar epithelium, or both. The relationship between the presence of HPV and neoplasia is, however, far from clear as sensitive techniques for the detection of HPV have shown that the virus may be present in normal epithelium and that it is more widely distributed in the population than is intra-epithelial neoplasia.

1.4.1   Cervical squamous intra-epithelial neoplasia (CIN)

Cervical squamous intra-epithelial neoplasia (CIN) is recognized by disturbances of cellular maturation and stratification, and cytological atypia. It is customarily graded according to its degree of cytoplasmic maturation (Anderson *et al.* 1991). It usually develops in the metaplastic squamous epithelium of the transformation zone. which lies on the ectocervix in the younger woman and in the endocervical canal in the older patient (Coleman and Evans 1988). The lesion may affect not only the surface epithelium but also the metaplastic squamous epithelium in the underlying crypts. Extension of the intra-epithelial lesion into the crypts can be distinguished from invasion by the regular, smooth contours of the *in situ* lesion in contrast with the somewhat irregular, jagged margins that characterize invasion, and the absence of a tissue response to the abnormal epithelium (Fig. 1.8). The area of epithelium affected by CIN may have irregular margins but is, initially, a single area. It can therefore be assumed that if the resection margins of the tissue removed during the treatment of CIN are free from disease that all the abnormality has been removed. This state may be altered by therapy if incomplete removal of a lesion leaves residual disease in more than one place. This is particularly worrying when the residual disease lies within the endocervical canal where direct observation is precluded. It is not uncommon, however, on initial examination of a lesion, to observe additional 'warty' patches on the vaginal epithelium

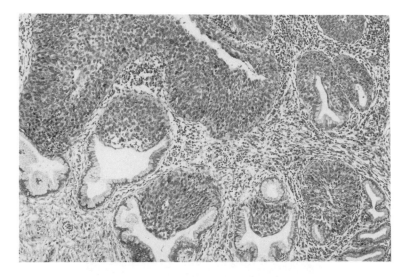

Fig. 1.8 Cervical intra-epithelial neoplasia (CIN) which extends into the crypts underlying the transformation zone. Note the smooth contours of the crypts and contrast them with the stromal invasion seen in Fig. 1.14.

which are separate from that on the cervix, or the cervical lesion may extend, in continuity, onto the vagina. These separate patches may be condylomatous or non-condylomatous and may or may not contain evidence of vaginal intra-epithelial neoplasia (VAIN). Vaginal lesions may also develop subsequently. Such findings cast doubt on the concept that carcinogenesis in this area is monoclonal (Burghardt 1992a). These separate foci may contain the same type of HPV or may contain different types.

CIN is customarily divided into three grades in Europe although suggestions for alternative grading systems have been proposed (Anderson *et al.* 1991).

The lesions range from a well differentiated intra-epithelial neoplasm, or CIN 1, to a poorly differentiated intra-epithelial neoplasm or CIN 3 with CIN 2 occupying an intermediate position. The differentiation of CIN is rarely uniform throughout the affected area, tending to be better on the outer, caudal part of the transformation zone, adjacent to the ectocervical squamous epithelium, and poorer adjacent to the endocervical epithelium on the inner, or medial, part of the transformation zone.

HPV types similar to those found in condylomatous lesions, and regarded as having a low risk of progression to invasive carcinoma, are identified in CIN, as well as types such as 16 and 18 which carry a higher risk of progression to invasive carcinoma (Franquemont *et al.* 1989: Willett *et al.* 1989). Although HPV types 16 and 18 are most commonly identified

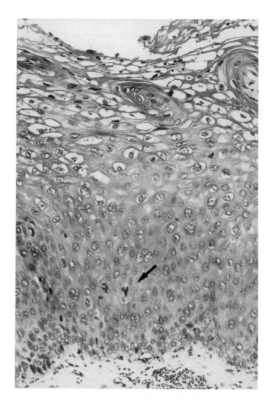

Fig. 1.9 A flat condyloma with an atypical mitosis (arrow). Its presence warrants the diagnosis of CIN 1 despite the absence of nuclear hyperchromasia and pleomorphism in the basal layers of the epithelium.

in CIN 2 and 3, such types also occur in CIN 1, flat condyloma, and even in women with no visible lesion. Thus identification of HPV type is of limited value in determining the appropriate management of a lesion although knowledge of its type may allow the clinician to give priority to certain individuals with low-grade lesions in whom treatment might otherwise have been delayed.

In CIN, nuclear abnormalities such as enlargement, pleomorphism, and hyperchromasia are present at all levels in the epithelium, including the basal layer. Atypical mitoses may be present in all grades (Fig. 1.9) (Buckley *et al.* 1982; Anderson *et al.* 1991). Normal mitotic figures vary in number and do not affect the diagnosis but the general degree of nuclear atypia is greater in CIN 3 than in CIN 1. In CIN I (previously known as mild dysplasia) cytoplasmic maturation occurs in the superfical two thirds of the epithelium (Fig. 1.10), in CIN 2 (previously known as moderate

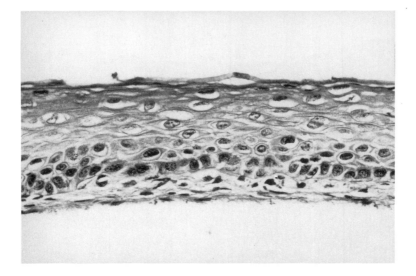

Fig. 1.10 Cervical intra-epithelial neoplasia Grade 1 (CIN 1). Nuclear hyperchromasia and pleomorphism is present in the basal third of the epithelium: the nuclear atypia persists to the surface of the epithelium but cytoplasmic maturation occurs in the outer two thirds.

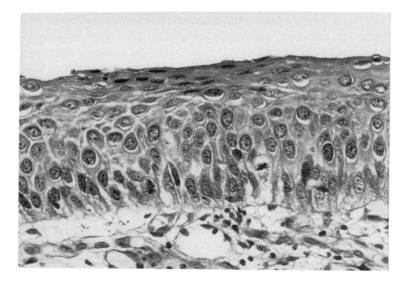

Fig. 1.11 Cervical intra-epithelial neoplasia Grade 2 (CIN 2). Nuclear enlargement and mild pleomorphism is present at all levels in the epithelium and cytoplasmic maturation occurs only in the outer half.

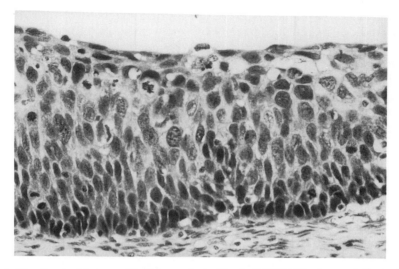

Fig. 1.12 Cervical intra-epithelial neoplasia Grade 3 (CIN 3). A population of cells with large, hyperchromatic, rather pleomorphic nuclei and very little cytoplasm occupies the full thickness of the epithelium.

dysplasia) cytoplasmic maturation commences in the middle third of the epithelium (Fig. 1.11) and in CIN 3 (including those abnormalities known previously as severe dysplasia and carcinoma *in situ*), cytoplasmic maturation, which is minimal, occurs in only part of the superficial third of the epithelium or is absent (Fig. 1.12). HPV-associated changes such as koilocytes and epithelial multinucleation are often present and are most conspicuous in CIN 1 and 2 and minimal or absent in CIN 3. This may be a reflection of the integration of the HPV although viral integration is less common than in carcinomas. The presence of 'warty' features in CIN makes histopathological grading of CIN more difficult and is a factor in the inter- and intra-observer variation in grading of CIN which has been reported.

1.4.2   The nomenclature of CIN

About 50 per cent of lesions diagnosed as CIN 1 will regress spontaneously and too early an intervention may result in the unnecessary treatment of women who are at little or no risk of developing carcinoma. There are, on the other hand, women with CIN 1 in whom the disease will persist or progress to carcinoma.

These difficulties, plus the fact that inter- and intra-observer differences are recognized in the grading of CIN, have fostered recommendations that histopathological opinion should relate more directly to the biological behaviour of CIN. It has been suggested that the three-tier histopathological grading of CIN should give way to a two-tier system, the new grades corresponding to those cases with a low risk of progression to carcinoma and those with a high risk.

Four different systems have been proposed, each of which aims to reduce the degree of diagnostic inconsistency between histopathologists, and to distinguish between low-grade lesions usually associated with HPV types 6 and 11, and associated with a low risk of progression to carcinoma, and those associated with HPV types 16 and 18 in which progression to carcinoma is more common.

The Bethesda system (Solomon 1989) suggests a division between 'low-grade intra-epithelial squamous lesions' (currently CIN 1 and flat condyloma) and 'high-grade intra-epithelial squamous lesions' (currently CIN 2 and CIN 3). Richart (1990), who first proposed the three-tier system in 1967, proposes a similar division but with slightly different terminology with 'low-grade CIN with HPV related changes' (currently CIN 1 and flat condyloma) and 'high-grade CIN' (currently CIN 2 and CIN 3). Ismail *et al.* (1989) propose that CIN 1 and HPV associated changes should be known as 'borderline CIN' and that only CIN 2 and CIN 3 should be known as 'CIN'. Finally, Robertson *et al.* (1989) suggest that the division should lie between 'low-grade CIN' (presently CIN 1 and CIN 2) and 'high-grade CIN' (presently CIN 3). It can be seen, therefore, that there is no agreement as to terminology or to the method of stratification. Indeed, the proposal to group CIN 2 with CIN 1 is not supported by viral studies, which show that HPV type 16 is found with some consistency in CIN 2 and 3 but with a lower frequency in CIN 1.

There are advantages to any system that gives a clear indication to the clinician as to the risk of an individual patient developing carcinoma but clinicians currently treat CIN 2 and CIN 3 similarly for the purposes of management and the new systems do not help in this respect. Moreover, the division of opinion as to where the separation into high and low risk categories should lie is confusing because there is no consensus as to where the division should lie and the reintroduction of a two-tier system may well encourage the misguided belief that intra-epithelial neoplasia of the cervix is a two-stage disease, a concept which is known to be fallacious and was one of the main reasons for replacing the old terminology of dysplasia and carcinoma *in situ* by that of CIN.

None of these proposals, therefore, solves the underlying problem. A histopathological report is an opinion that depends upon interpretation and until such time as there is an objective way of assessing intra-epithelial changes it will remain so. We can reduce inter-observer variation by ensuring adequate training of histopathologists but we cannot completely abolish it. Moreover, none of the suggestions helps in the case of the individual patient. Even the identification of HPV type will not help in those patients in whom there is morphological CIN 3 with so-called low-risk virus types or no detectable lesion in the presence of high-risk virus types. It is for these reasons that the Working Party set up by the National Coordinating Network of the NHS Cervical Screening Programme and the British Society for Clinical Cytology proposed that, for the time being, in the UK we would continue to use the three-tier system of grading that is in current use (Anderson *et al.* 1991).

1.4.3   Cervical glandular intra-epithelial neoplasia (CGIN)

Cervical glandular intra-epithelial neoplasia, the term incorporating 'glandular atypia' and 'adenocarcinoma *in situ*', also most commonly develops on the transformation zone. It thus tends to lie on the ectocervix in younger women and within the endocervical canal in older women, in the same area of the cervix as squamous intra-epithelial neoplasia with which it is often associated. There is supportive evidence for the role of HPV 18 in the aetiology of CGIN (Wells 1992).

Both the surface epithelium and the underlying crypts can be affected. In the typical lesion (Fig. 1.13) the epithelium is stratified, there is a reduction in intracytoplasmic mucin, and there is an increase in nucleo-cytoplasmic ratios. The nuclei are hyperchromatic, pleomorphic, to a variable degree, and nucleoli (which may be multiple and large) may be seen. In the less-common form of the disease, the cells are of intestinal type, of either goblet cell or signet ring form. The junction between the abnormal epithelium and the adjacent normal columnar epithelium is invariably abrupt. In all but the most minor lesions glandular morphology is abnormal with complex infolding, outpouchings or budding, intraluminal papillary projections, and epithelial bridge formation. Glandular crowding may be present.

Criteria for grading CGIN are less well established than are the criteria for grading CIN but CGIN 3 corresponds to adenocarcinoma *in situ* and CGIN 1 and 2 correspond to lesser degrees of cytological and glandular morphological abnormality. Rarely, CGIN may extend, synchronously or following treatment of the cervical lesion, to the vagina. CGIN of clear cell type, occurring in women with vaginal adenosis, may also follow this pattern, although to the best of my knowledge there is no evidence that this form of the disease is HPV-associated.

There is less knowledge about the relationship of CGIN to invasive adenocarcinoma of the cervix than about CIN and squamous carcinoma of the cervix although it is known that at least some of the lesions progress to carcinoma.

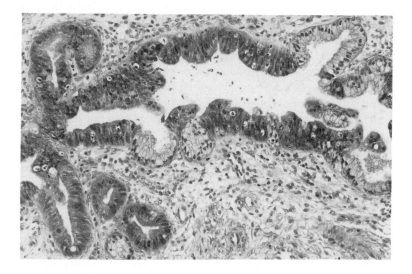

Fig. 1.13 Cervical glandular intra-epithelial neoplasia (CGIN). The crypt is lined partly by normal mucin-secreting epithelium (top right) and partly by epithelium with the features of CGIN. The latter is stratified, the cells have high nucleo-cytoplasmic ratios, the nuclei are darkly staining and contain mitoses, and there is little mucin secretion.

In an uncommon form of the disease, adenocarcinoma *in situ* develops in an area of endometrial metaplasia within the endocervical canal. Such lesions may be associated with the presence of an invasive endometrioid adenocarcinoma but the evidence for an association with this form of CGIN and HPV has not been established.

1.5   Carcinoma of the cervix

The majority of cervical carcinomas develop from an abnormal transformation zone. They tend to lie, therefore, on the ectocervix in the young women and in the endocervical canal in the older woman, the position of the transformation zone determining the position of the tumour. The carcinomas may be exophytic or endophytic, those on the ectocervix being more commonly exophytic and those in the canal more commonly endophytic, expanding the tissues and producing the typical barrel-shaped cervix. This has some clinical importance in that exophytic tumours on the ectocervix are less likely to have extended to the adjacent tissues and organs than endophytic tumours of similar size, and are less likely to have metastasized.

Cervical carcinomas spread locally into the cervical stroma, the para-cervical and parametrial tissues, the body of the uterus, the vagina, and, late in the course of the disease, to the bladder and rectum. Lymphatic permeation in the cervical stroma may be seen even when the tumour is still of low volume and hence pelvic lymph node metastases may be found even in women who appear, at clinical examination, to have early carcinoma. It is impossible, therefore, to equate small carcinoma with early carcinoma. Blood-borne spread and distant metastases are a late manifestation of the disease.

It is usual to divide the invasive lesions of the cervix into two major categories. The first of these are those termed micro-invasive and the second are the frankly invasive carcinomas.

1.5.1   Micro-invasive carcinoma

A micro-invasive squamous carcinoma is small, and can be diagnosed only by histological means (Lowe 1992). It offers the possibility of relatively conservative treatment because of the low, but not absent, risk of metastatic disease. The definition and management of such cases is the subject of controversy and those definitions using the depth of invasion only as the major criterion are now regarded as being rather dangerous and unsuitable as a basis for determining a plan of management (Burghardt 1992b). Micro-invasive carcinoma is defined by the International Federation of Gynecology and Obstetrics as Stage IA (FIGO 1986) and two categories are recognized, early stromal invasion and microcarcinoma. Early stromal invasion (FIGO Stage Ia1) is recognized by the presence of non-confluent buds of neoplastic cells infiltrating into the stroma from the basal layer of an epithelium with the features of CIN or, apparently separate foci of invasive cells lying no more than 1 mm from the basement membrane of either a surface or crypt epithelium in which there are features of CIN (Fig. 1.14). There is often greater cytoplasmic maturation than in the intra-epithelial component and as a consequence the cytoplasm is eosinophilic. Such lesions can be treated in the same way as CIN, but if early stromal invasion has been detected on an initial punch biopsy, cone biopsy is the treatment of choice so that histopathological examination can exclude the presence of a more deeply invasive tumour. The cone biopsy is regarded as having provided adequate therapy for lesions of this type if all invasive and intra-epithelial neoplasia has been completely excised.

Microcarcinoma (Stage Ia2) is described as a measurable confluent tumour up to 5 mm deep, measured from the base of the epithelium from which it arises, whether crypt or surface, and with a horizontal spread of no more than 7 mm (FIGO 1986). Permeation of endothelial lined spaces is ignored in this definition. Stage Ia2 lesions, as defined in this manner, cannot all be safely treated only by cone biopsy. The Committee of Nomenclature of

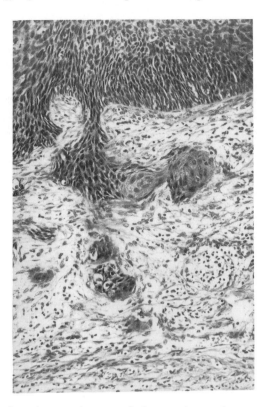

Fig. 1.14 Micro-invasive carcinoma of the cervix: early stromal invasion. An epithelium with the features of CIN 3 lies at the top of the illustration and from its base there arise tongues of invading tumour the cells of which have a greater quantity of pale cytoplasm than the cells in the CIN from which it arises. There is a lymphocytic infiltrate in the surrounding stroma.

the Society of Gynecologic Oncology (SGO) (Seski *et al.* 1977) suggested reducing the depth of invasion to 3 mm or less, and excluded lesions in which there is also vascular permeation. Even this, however, does not ensure freedom from the risk of metastases yet may result in unnecessarily radical treatment for some women. Definitions of microinvasive carcinoma should, therefore, consider tumour volume, vascular permeation, and, although it has yet to be established in a large prospective study, the expression of growth factors.

The term microinvasive carcinoma can be applied to adenosquamous carcinomas as well as to squamous carcinomas but no clearly defined criteria have been established for the diagnosis of microadenocarcinoma. Attention has, however, been drawn to the possibility that such entities may exist (Rollason *et al.* 1989; Lowe 1992) (Fig. 1.15).

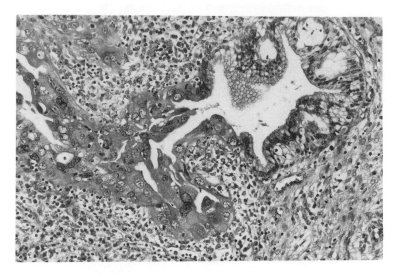

Fig. 1.15 Micro-invasive adenocarcinoma. The crypt (to the upper right) is lined, in its lower part, by an epithelium with the features of CGIN and from it (at the lower left) there arises a focus of superficially invasive adenocarcinoma.

1.5.2   Invasive carcinoma

Squamous carcinoma

Squamous carcinomas constitute 70 to 78 per cent of cervical malignancies (Buckley and Fox 1992). They may be well-differentiated (large cell tumours showing well-marked keratinization), moderately differentiated (large cell tumours with focal keratinization), or poorly differentiated (large and small cell tumours with minimal evidence of keratinization). The majority of these neoplasms are moderately or poorly differentiated, only about 10 per cent being well differentiated. Integrated and episomal HPV types 16 and 18 have been detected in squamous carcinoma of the cervix and there may be histological evidence of its presence in the form of KA.

The well-differentiated carcinomas grow in bands or discrete islands whilst less-well-differentiated neoplasms grow in an infiltrative pattern or form solid sheets. The well-differentiated carcinomas are characterized by intercellular bridges and well-formed epithelial pearls (Fig. 1.16).

A rare form of exceptionally well-differentiated squamous carcinoma is the verrucous carcinomas in which the histological features closely resemble a *condyloma acuminatum*. HPV type 6 has been isolated from such neoplasms and KA is a common histological feature. The tumours are often misinterpreted as condylomata when first biopsied and it is only

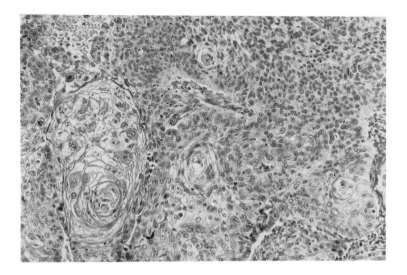

Fig. 1.16 Well differentiated squamous carcinoma. The tumour forms concentric arrangements of cells which mature towards their centres to form epithelial pearls.

their locally agressive behaviour and tendency to recur that draws attention to their malignant nature.

Moderately differentiated squamous carcinoma shows a greater degree of cellular pleomorphism, higher nucleo-cytoplasmic ratios and more frequent mitoses. Intercellular bridges are scanty, ill-formed or absent: epithelial pearls are rarely seen but individually keratinized, dyskeratotic cells, recognizable by their densely eosinophilic cytoplasm, occur singly or in small groups.

Poorly differentiated squamous carcinomas (Fig. 1.17) are often diagnosed simply because their growth pattern or constituent cells are similar to those of a squamous neoplasm. The diagnosis should not, however, be made on morphological grounds alone in the absence of some evidence of squamous differentiation, such as occasional dyskeratotic cells, or the demonstration of cytokeratin subtype by immunohistochemistry. Mucin secretion and glandular differentiation should also be excluded (Buckley *et al.* 1988).

Contradictory results have been obtained in respect of the importance of the levels of epidermal growth factor receptor (EGF-R), some reporting an increased risk of lymph node metastases and recurrence or death from disease irrespective of the clincal stage of the disease (Pfeiffer *et al.* 1989) and others finding no relationship (Hayashi *et al.* 1991). Overexpression of c-myc proto-oncogene is associated with an increased risk of relapse

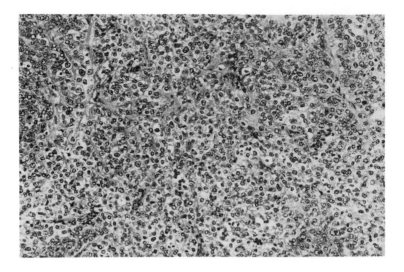

Fig. 1.17 Poorly differentiated, non-keratinizing squamous carcinoma. The cells grow as solid sheets. Note the similarity to the poorly differentiated adenocarcinoma seen in Fig. 1.20.

(Bourhis *et al.* 1990), and a greater tendency to develop extrapelvic metastases (Sowani *et al.* 1989) whilst preliminary data suggest that expression of ras oncogene product p21 is associated with an increased risk of nodal metastases (Hayashi *et al.* 1991).

Adenosquamous carcinoma

Adenosquamous carcinoma (Fig. 1.18) often develops from CIN and may be well, moderately, or poorly differentiated. These tumours show a greater tendency to metastasize widely, even when the lesion in the cervix is small, and are disproportionately common in women under the age of 40 years (Buckley *et al.* 1988).

It is our experience that those tumours in which C-erbB-2 and EGFR are identified immunohistochemically are more likely to have a poor outcome, the correlation being most marked when there are no lymph node metastases at the time of diagnosis (Hale *et al.* 1992; Hale *et al.* 1993).

Adenocarcinoma

Adenocarcinomas constitute between 12 and 18.6 per cent of malignant cervical neoplasms (Buckley and Fox 1992), and the incidence is reported to be increasing. They cannot be distinguished grossly from squamous

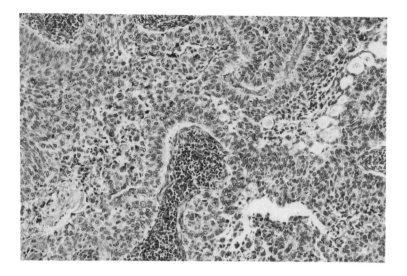

Fig. 1.18 Poorly differentiated adenosquamous carcinoma. To the lower left, the tumour forms an abortive squamous epithelial pearl and to the upper right, there are small glandular structures.

carcinomas, having a similar morphology and site of origin in the cervix. HPV types 16 and 18 have been identified in different types of adeno-carcinomas of the cervix by means of *in situ* hybridization (Wells 1992) but type 18 is more common than in squamous carcinoma. CIN and/or CGIN may be present in the epithelium adjacent to any of the main adenocarcinomatous tumour types.

   The prognosis for women with adenocarcinoma of the cervix is significantly worse than for those with squamous carcinoma (Brown 1992), particularly when nodal metastases are present (Hale *et al.* 1991). Adeno-carcinomas are of several different types. The majority are composed of tissue resembling that of the normal endocervix and may be very well differentiated, so-called minimal deviation carcinoma (Fig. 1.19), or are more typical endocervical carcinomas. They develop most commonly from the columnar epithelium of an ectopy, or more correctly from an adenocar-cinoma *in situ* or CGIN which has formed on the cervical ectopy. Other cervical adenocarcinomas are characterized by the presence of intestinal epithelium, serous epithelium resembling that of the fallopian tube or endometrioid differentiation. The latter are the exception to the rule that these tumours form on the cervical ectopy. They develop in the older woman and are more commonly found in the endocervical canal. Their clinical correlates also more closely resemble those of endometrial carcinoma.

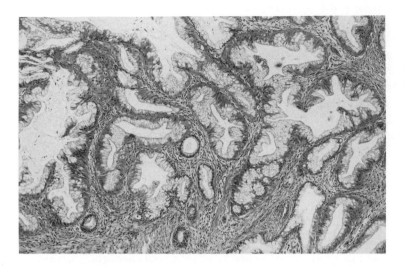

Fig. 1.19 Minimal deviation adenocarcinoma. The tumour is composed of well differentiated glandular structures which resemble normal endocervical crypts. There is, as the name suggests, minimal cytological atypia in the epithelium.

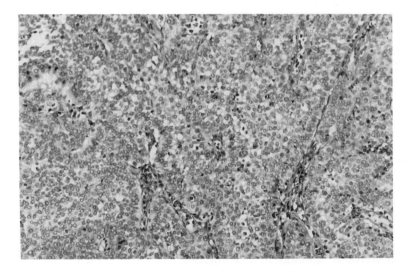

Fig. 1.20 Poorly differentiated adenocarcinoma. The tumour cells form solid sheets. The correct nature of this neoplasm would not have been determined without the use of histochemical tests to demonstrate the presence of intracytoplasmic mucus. Note its similarity to the squamous carcinoma seen in Fig. 1.17.

The proportion of adenocarcinomas is often underestimated for want of careful histopathological evaluation. Since as adenocarcinomas become less well differentiated, they tend to more closely resemble poorly differentiated squamous carcinoma from which they can be distinguished only by the presence of mucin (Fig. 1.20).

Adenocarcinomas also exhibit neuroendocrine differentiation and there may, therefore, be systemic manifestations of their presence. HPV has been identified even in tumours of this type. It is our experience that adenocarcinomas are not more likely than squamous carcinoma to metastasize but once metastases have developed the outlook is grim.

1.6 Diagnostic techniques

1.6.1 The cervical smear test

This text has dealt with the recognition and detection of HPV, intraepithelial and invasive neoplasia in tissue sections but in most cases the presence of HPV and CIN is first suspected following the recognition, in a cervical smear, of abnormal cells.

The cervical smear test was designed as a screening test for the detection of squamous intra-epithelial neoplasia and is based on the fact that the nuclear abnormalities of CIN are present throughout the whole thickness of the epithelium and can thus be detected in cells scraped from the surface of the lesion. The chance of detecting CIN is also enhanced by the fact that there tends to be poor cellular adhesion between the neoplastic cells and they are thus more readily removed during the scraping process. The chances of their detection is, however, diminished by a poorly taken, unrepresentive smear, the withdrawal of the abnormal transformation zone to within the endocervical canal and a small lesion. The test also allows the detection of CGIN but there are greater difficulties in interpreting columnar cell changes than there are in interpreting squamous epithelial changes.

Although the test was designed to detect intra-epithelial neoplasia, it may also detect wart virus infection. Such infections are suggested by the presence of KA, multinucleated epithelial cells, cells with rather enlarged minimally atypical nuclei, and cells with dense hyperchromatic nuclei and densely eosinophilic cytoplasm which have been shed from an area of parakeratosis. HPV can be identified in cervical scrape material using a variety of techniques but it is less consistently positive than similar tests on a biopsy from the same lesion or patient.

The cervical smear test may also identify the presence of a carcinoma although this is not its primary function, and detection of a cervical carcinoma represents a failure of the screening programme which, by identifying and allowing treatment of the intra-epithelial lesion, should prevent the development of carcinoma. It is, nonetheless, the means whereby a proportion of carcinomas are first identified.

1.6.2   Colposcopic examination

Colposcopic examination of the cervix involves direct examination of the cervix under magnification and allows directed biopsy of abnormal areas. It is designed to detect the source of the cytological abnormality seen in the smear. The technique is enhanced by the application of Lugol's iodine (to detect glycogen), weak acetic acid (to identify areas of epithelial abnormality), and viewing the cervix through a green filter to identify the vascular pattern which can be seen through the epithelium and distortion of which is a useful indicator of the presence of CIN. The information which is obtained from this technique depends heavily upon the expertise of the operator.

Prompt colposcopic assessment is indicated when there is moderate or severe dyskaryosis, and can be carried out as soon as is convenient when there is persistent mild dyskaryosis or borderline changes in the smears. Urgent colposcopic evaluation is required if there is severe dyskaryosis, suggesting the possibility of carcinoma.

Although it is usual to regard areas which are aceto-white, Schiller positive (lacking glycogen), and having an abnormal vascular pattern as CIN, in fact, none of these changes is specific for CIN. For example, metaplastic squamous epithelium is often less well glycogenated than the original squamous epithelium of the ectocervix, immature metaplastic squamous epithelium appears aceto-white, and an abnormal vascular pattern is frequently observed in a condylomatous lesion.

Colposcopic biopsy

Should the colposcopist identify an abnormal area, a punch biopsy will be taken. This is usually no more than 0.5 cm in diameter but when taken with care may allow precise correlation between the smear and the histological appearances. The biopsy is usually examined at several levels to ensure that the range of abnormalities has been fully explored. This is particularly important as the finding of even early stromal invasion demands that the patient be treated by cone biopsy rather than local ablation.

The colposcopic biopsy often, but not invariably, includes part of the stroma of the transformation zone, the surface epithelium and part of the underlying crypts. It is usual to find a range of epithelial abnormalities even in such a small biopsy and the abnormality may be limited to one or two of the several histological sections examined.

More recently there has been a tendency to carry out a diagnostic and therapeutic process at the first colposcopic examination and remove the whole of the transformation zone with a diathermy loop rather than sample the abnormal transformation zone. This has some advantages, in that the tissue can be examined more thoroughly than in a simple punch biopsy, and the whole of the transformation zone may be removed. There are, however, in my experience, disadvantages which include the fact that that a number of women will be subjected to excision biopsy when the nature of their lesion did not require such therapy and there may be such severe coagulation artifact in the biopsy that interpretation of the tissue may be difficult, or even impossible. It is yet another technique that depends heavily upon the skill of the operator.

Should the colposcopist be unable to identify any abnormality on examination of the cervix, the lesion may lie in the vagina or within the endocervical canal. One of the most important parts of the colposcopic examination is the identification of the squamocolumnar junction. If this lies beyond the vision of the operator, in the endocervical canal, and the source of the abnormal cells cannot be seen, a cone biopsy may be required for evaluation of the cervix. A cone biopsy is also required if a colposcopic biopsy reveals any evidence of stromal invasion and if the biopsy fails to reveal the source of the abnormal cells seen in the cervical biopsy.

1.6.3   Cone biopsy

A cone biopsy is, as its name suggests, a conical or pyramidal piece of tissue with its base on the ectocervix around and including the external os and its apex extending into the endocervical canal. It contains a segment of the endocervical canal and it is intended to remove the entire abnormal transformation zone. It is examined to ensure that the abnormality has been completely removed and that there is no evidence of invasive tumour.

The pathologist should be able, following examination of a colposcopic punch biopsy, to determine whether the colposcopist has found a lesion explaining the cytological abnormality and exclude invasion in that area. The loop biopsy or cone biopsy is both therapeutic and diagnostic. It should determine the range of abnormality present, determine whether excision of the transformation zone is complete or not, determine whether all abnormal epithelium has been removed, and finally, exclude the presence of invasion.

Should the cytological examination, the biopsy, or the colposcopic examination raise the possibility that there is an invasive lesion, a cone biopsy is mandatory to determine the site and degree of invasion. The management of an invasive lesion depends upon the stage and extent of the carcinoma and not upon the grade or histological type.

Follow-up of patients who have had treatment of CIN is usually by repeat cervical smears and colposcopic examination as indicated by the cytological findings. It is usual for these to be repeated more frequently in the year following the treatment and yearly thereafter for about five years. The follow-up of women who have been treated for CIN has become a burden to the system and in general people now feel more confident about returning women to routine, rather than special, follow-up.

References

Anderson, M. C., Brown, C. L., Buckley, C. H., Fox, H., Jenkins, D. G., Lowe, D. G. *et al.* (1991). Current views on cervical intra-epithelial neoplasia. *Journal of Clinical Pathology*, **44**, 969–78.

Bourhis, J., Le, M. G., Barrois, M., Gerbaulet, A. J. (1990). Prognostic value of c-myc proto-oncogene overexpression in early invasive carcinoma of the cervix. *Journal of Clinical Oncology*, **8**, 1789–96.

Brown, L. J. R. (1992). Abnormalities of the glandular epithelium of the endocervix. In *Advances in gynaecological pathology* (ed. D. Lowe and H. Fox), pp. 163–89. Churchill Livingstone, Edinburgh.

Buckley, C. H. and Fox, H. (1992). Pathology of clinical invasive carcinoma of cervix. In *Gynecologic oncology: fundamental principles and practice* (2nd edn) (ed. M. Coppleson), pp. 649–62. Churchill Livingstone, Edinburgh.

Buckley, C. H., Butler, E. B., and Fox, H. (1982). Cervical intra-epithelial neoplasia. *Journal of Clinical Pathology*, **35**, 1–13.

Buckley, C. H., Beards, C. S., and Fox, H. (1988). Pathological prognostic indicators in cervical cancer with particular reference to patients under the age of 40 years. *British Journal of Obstetrics and Gynaecology*, **95**, 47–56.

Burghardt, E. (1992a). Is cervical cancer monoclonal? *Lancet*, **340**, 1543–4.

Burghardt, E. (1992b). Pathology of early invasive squamous and glandular carcinoma of the cervix (FIGO Stage Ia). In *Gynecologic oncology: fundamental principles and practice* (2nd edn) (ed. M. Coppleson), pp. 609–29. Churchill Livingstone, Edinburgh.

Coleman, D. V. and Evans, D. M. D. (1988). *Biopsy pathology and cytology of the cervix*. Chapman and Hall, London.

FIGO 1986 Cancer Committee. Staging announcement. *Gynecological Oncology*, **25**, 383–85.

Franquemont, D. W., Ward, B. E., Andersen, W. A., and Crum, C. P. (1989). Prediction of "high-risk" cervical papillomavirus infection by biopsy morphology. *American Journal of Clinical Pathology*, **92**, 577–92.

Hale, R. J., Wilcox, F. L., Buckley, C. H., Tindall, V. R., Ryder, W. D. J., and Logue, J. P. (1991). Prognostic factors in uterine cervical carcinoma: a clinicopathological analysis. *International Journal of Gynecological Pathology*, **1**, 19–23.

Hale, R. J., Buckley, C. H., Fox, H., and Williams, J. (1992). Prognostic value of c-erbB-2 expression in uterine cervical carcinoma. *Journal of Clinical Pathology*, **45**, 594–6.

Hale, R. J., Buckley, C. H., Gullick W. J., Fox, H., Williams, J., and Wilcox, F. L. (1993). Prognostic value of epidermal growth factor receptor expression in cervical carcinoma. *Journal of Clinical Pathology*, **46**, 149–53.

Hayashi, Y., Hachisuga, T., Iwasaki, T., Fukuda, K., Okuma, Y., Yokoyama, M. *et al.* (1991). Expression of ras oncogene product and EGF receptor in cervical squamous carcinomas and its relationship to lymph node involvement. *Gynecologic Oncology*, **40**, 147–51.

Ismail, S. M., Colclough, A. B., Dinnen, J. S. Eakins, D., Evans, D. M. D., Gradwell, E. *et al.* (1989). Observer variation in histopathological diagnosis and grading of cervical intra-epithelial neoplasia. *British Medical Journal*, **298**, 707–10.

Lowe, D. (1992). Micro-invasive carcinoma of the lower female genital tract. In *Advances in gynaecological pathology*. (ed. D. Lowe and H. Fox), pp. 145–62. Churchill Livingstone, Edinburgh.

Pfeiffer, D., Stellwag, B., Pfeiffer, A., Borlinghaus, P., Meier, W., and Scheidel, P. (1989). Clinical implications of the epidermal growth factor receptor in the squamous cell carcinoma of the uterine cervix. *Gynecologic Oncology*, **33**, 146–50.

Richart, R. M. (1990). A modified terminology for cervical intra-epithelial neoplasia. *Obstetrics and Gynecology*, **75**, 131–33.

Robertson, A. J., Anderson, J. M., Swanson Beck, J., Burnett, R. A., Howatson, S. R., Lee, F. D. *et al.* (1989). Observer variability in histopathological reporting of cervical biopsy specimens. *Journal of Clinical Pathology*, **42**, 231–38.

Rollason, T. P., Cullimore, J., and Bradgate, M. G. (1989). A suggested columnar cell morphological equivalent of squamous carcinoma *in situ* with early stromal invasion. *International Journal of Gynecological Pathology*, **8**, 230–36.

Seski, J. C., Murray, R. A., and Morley, G. (1977). Microinvasive squamous carcinoma of the cervix: definition, histologic analysis, late results of treatment. *Obstetrics and Gynecology*, **50**, 410–14.

Solomon, D. (1989). The 1988 Bethesda system for reporting cervical/vaginal cytological diagnoses. *Acta Cytologica*, **33**, 567–74.

Sowani, A., Ong, G., Dische, S. Quinn, C., White, J., Soutter, P. *et al.* (1989). C-myc oncogene expression and clinical outome in carcinoma of the cervix. *Molecular and Cellular Probes*, **3**, 117–23.

Wells, M. (1992). Human papillomavirus associated lesions of the lower female genital tract. In *Advances in Gynaecological Pathology* (ed. D. Lowe and H. Fox), pp. 79–97. Churchill Livingstone, Edinburgh.

Willett, G. D., Kurman, R. J., Reid, R. Greenberg, M., Bennet-Jenson, A. and Lorincz, A. T. (1989). Correlation of the histologic appearance of intra-epithelial neoplasia of the cervix with human papillomavirus types: emphasis on low grade lesions including so-called flat condyloma. *International Journal of Gynecological Pathology*, **8**, 18–25.

2 Molecular genetics of human papillomaviruses

JOHN R. ARRAND

2.1 Introduction

It is an interesting outcome of the age of molecular biology that one can contemplate describing the genetics of an organism when the actual beast itself has not been encountered in a free-living, natural state. Yet this is exactly the situation which pertains to several types of human papillomaviruses. It is only very recently that some of the most widely studied papilloma 'viruses' have actually been observed as fully formed particles but even so only *in vitro* (Sterling *et al.* 1990). Nevertheless, by virtue of genetic manipulation technology a great deal is known about this fascinating and clinically important genus of the family *Papovaviridae*.

This chapter summarizes, with particular reference to HPV types associated with cervical lesions, some of the findings in relation to the genome structure and transcription of papillomaviruses, functions of individual gene products, and the genetic relationships both within and between types.

2.2 Genome structure and organization

As alluded to above it is often impossible to detect or isolate HPV particles in or from their associated lesions. In those lesions from which virus particles could be isolated in workable quantity, for example skin warts on humans or cattle (containing HPV-1 or BPV-1, respectively) the viral genome was found to be a double stranded circular DNA molecule. However, in most types of papillomavirus-associated lesion, virus DNA is present intracellularly, frequently as an extrachromosomal episome and occasionally, for example, in some carcinomas, integrated within the host chromosomes. This viral DNA can therefore be molecularly cloned and characterized. HPVs are classified on the basis of their host range and DNA sequence homology; the definition of a distinct type being that, on reassociation analysis in solution, its DNA must exhibit less than 50 per cent homology with any other known type from that host species. This is in fact a more rigorous criterion than that which applies to many other types of viruses which are distinguished on, for example, serological relationships. Human

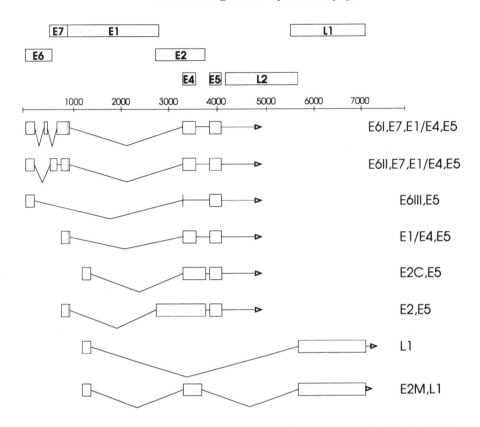

Fig. 2.1 Organisation of the HPV16 genome and arrangement of spliced mRNAs. At the top the HPV16 genome is represented in a linear fashion by the horizontal line and the positions of the various open reading frames are depicted as open boxes. The scale is in nucleotide pairs. Below the map is shown the arrangement of mRNA species which have been mapped to the genome. The open boxes represent potential coding regions whilst splices are indicated by the angled lines. The coding potential of each species is shown on the right.

adenovirus serotypes 1 to 31 would be regarded as consisting of only five types if the papillomavirus criteria were employed in their case (Green *et al.* 1979).

Currently at least seventy different HPV genotypes have been described (E.-M. de Villiers, personal communication) together with several subtypes. The complete DNA sequences of several HPVs from a variety of clinical sources have been determined, together with those of papillomaviruses of other hosts, for example cattle, rabbit, and chaffinch. The Genbank database (release 77) lists complete sequences for 23 papillomavirus types and sequences for several additional HPVs have been determined (quoted in Chan *et al.*

1992b). In all cases the genome is approximately 8000 base pairs in length. Analysis of these sequences for potential open reading frames (ORFs) revealed a remarkable consistency in the overall genetic organization of the DNA from all types and species. This 'classical' physical map of papillomaviruses is shown in Fig. 2.1 and consists of a number of open reading frames and an approximately 1kb non-coding region. The so-called 'early' (E) ORFs encode proteins involved in DNA replication, transcription, and cellular transformation whilst the 'late' (L) ORFs specify the viral capsid proteins. In BPV eight early ORFs were identified. These generally have counterparts in other papillomaviruses with the exceptions of E3 and E8. E3 is now generally accepted as being a spurious reading frame which does not actually encode protein (Hermonat and Howley, 1987) whilst E8 seems to be involved in BPV replication (M. Lusky, quoted in DiMaio and Neary, 1990). There is not an E8 homologue in HPV.

2.3   Transcription

Whilst the simplistic identification of the coding potential of these viruses based on examination of their DNA sequences has proved to be a very fruitful exercise in forming the basis of functional analysis, the actual protein products are potentially more complex due to various RNA splicing events. In contrast to polyomaviruses (the other genus within the *Papovaviridae*), papillomavirus genetic information is transcribed and translated in one direction from only one strand of the DNA. Studies of cDNA structure have been performed by various laboratories and a summary of the results obtained for HPV-16 is depicted in Fig. 2.1. From these data several generalizations can be made:

(1) The splicing pattern is complex and generates a multiplicity of different mRNA species;

(2) some ORFs (e.g. E6 and E2) are represented to different extents in different messages;

(3) some ORFs appear to be expressed as fusion proteins of portions of two ORFs (e.g. E1/E4);

(4) many mRNAs are polycistronic.

The products of the E6 and E7 genes appear to play pivotal roles in papillomavirus-associated oncogenesis, in terms of both establishment and maintenance (see Chapter 5) and for this reason the transcription pattern of these genes has been examined with great interest. The overall conclusions from studies of non-malignant and malignant cell lines or of pre-malignant and malignant tumours and metastases suggest that variety in splicing patterns or RNA transcripts is not involved in HPV16-associated malignant progression (Sherman *et al.* 1992).

The generalizations made above are valid for other HPV types but the detailed transcriptional patterns are often not identical. For example, Smotkin *et al.* (1989) showed differences in promoter usage and splicing of mRNA in the E6 and E7 regions of the nononcogenic (types 6 and 11) and oncogenic (type 16) genital HPVs. The non-oncogenic types do not have splicing signals for the formation of the E6* products. It is suggestive that this and potential differences in the efficiency of internal reinitiation of translation required to generate the E7 protein may have some influence on the oncogenicity of the different types.

Functional bicistronic mRNA is very rare in eukaryotes. Of the few known cellular genes which are translated from such mRNAs, about 50 per cent are proto-oncogenes (Kozak 1987). Picornaviruses (Jackson *et al.* 1990) utilize internal ribosomal entry sites and Epstein–Barr virus (Wang *et al.* 1987) also appears to produce active polycistronic messages. Translational initiation at the internal AUG on the downstream coding region of these bicistronic RNAs is not compatible with current thinking on the mechanism of eukaryotic protein synthesis (Kozak 1989). Further work is required to resolve these issues.

2.4   Functions of HPV-encoded polypeptides

Because of the difficulties of propagating HPV *in vitro*, a large proportion of functional studies on the various papillomavirus proteins have been performed using BPV as the workable system of choice. It is an assumption that, because of the tight genetic homologies throughout the papillomavirus group, the basic properties of a given ORF from one virus will also be pertinent to other types. The following summary will, as far as possible, concentrate on data obtained from HPV. The E6 and E7 ORFs are considered in detail in Chapter 5 and therefore are not dealt with here.

2.4.1   E1

Studies using the BPV system have established that E1 is absolutely required for virus DNA replication. Inactivation of the E1 ORF by mutagenesis (frameshift, deletion, or insertion) results in integration of the viral DNA into the host chromosomal sequences with concomitant loss of the persistent episomal form of BPV DNA. Two replication functions have been ascribed to E1, the first being a modulator (E1-M) function encoded by the first one third of the ORF, whilst the second, specified by the remainder of the coding sequence, is a positive replicative function (E1-R). The entire ORF also appears to be involved in transcriptional repression. The E1-M function is required to maintain the BPV1 episome at constant copy number in transformed mouse C127 cells. HPV11-containing cells express a spliced mRNA fusing the E1M domain to the C-terminal portion of E2 (E1M^E2). The product of this message exhibited properties consistent with a role in modulation of replication (Chiang *et al.* 1991).

Nucleotide sequence comparisons have revealed regions of homology between a region of E1 towards its C-terminus and the ATPase active site of SV40 and Polyoma virus large T-antigens. Similar comparisons also suggested that E1 may have helicase activity and this prediction has recently been functionally confirmed (Yang *et al.* 1993).

Recently the E1 protein from HPV11 has been expressed from a baculovirus vector (Bream *et al.* 1993) and shown to exhibit properties in common with those previously defined for the BPV analogue. This recombinant HPV11 E1 forms a heteromeric complex with HPV11 E2, binds to DNA sequences which contain the viral origin of replication, and possesses ATPase and GTPase enzymatic activity. This latter property may be part of an energy-generating system for the ATP-dependent helicase function.

HPV16 E1 may have a role in repression of immortalizing potential since full-length DNA containing a non-functional E1 ORF is more efficient at immortalization of primary keratinocytes than is wild type DNA (Romanczuk and Howley 1992).

2.4.2   E2

E2 is a complex ORF which, like E1, has been studied principally in the BPV system. It is required for DNA replication in conjunction with its heteromeric partner E1. Like E1, mutations which inactivate E2 result in integration of viral DNA and loss of ability of the genome to be maintained as an episome. The E2 protein recognizes and binds to the target sequence $ACCN_6GGT$ which occurs as a conserved motif within the origins of replication of many papillomaviruses.

In addition to its role in replication E2 is also involved in transcriptional regulation. The full-length protein has transactivating functions on enhancer and promoter sequences whilst shorter forms derived from alternatively spliced mRNAs (E2C in Fig. 2.1) are transcriptional repressors.

A third important effect of BPV1 E2 is its effect on the transforming potential of the virus DNA. Although E2 itself cannot induce focus formation in mouse C127 cells, E2 mutants affect focus forming efficiency of the whole viral genome.

This complexity of functions ascribed to E2 of BPV1 can be manifested in at least four different phenotypes depending on the nature of mutation (DiMaio and Neary, 1990).

1. Mutants in which the defect is upstream of the splice acceptor site are compromised in their abilities to form foci, replicate, and transactivate. However, the defects can be complemented by wild-type E2.

2. Mutations downstream of the splice acceptor result in similar defects but in this case the flaw in transforming ability is non-complementable.

3. Deletions at the 3′ end of the coding sequence have normal focus-forming ability but are not fully competent at transactivation and will not support episomal replication.

4. A mutation specifically rendering the splice acceptor inactive is fully able to transactivate, is reduced in replicative ability, but fully competent at focus formation.

In the case of the human viruses, E2 clearly has an effect on the process of immortalization/transformation but the precise mechanism is still uncertain. Romanczuk and Howley (1992) describe experiments which indicate that E2-disrupted HPV16 DNA is more efficient at immortalization of primary human keratinocytes than is wild type DNA. On the other hand Storey *et al.* (1992) found that HPV16 DNA containing a mutant E2 ORF was lacking in immortalizing activity. Münger *et al.* (1989) complete the variations by their finding that defective E2 has no effect on immortalizing potential!

2.4.3 E4

In spite of its genomic position within the early region of the papillomavirus genome the E4 ORF appears to be a late protein in the sense that it accumulates intracellularly along with the virion structural proteins L1 and L2. Nevertheless it does not appear to be a component of the virus particle. It is, however, in some cases a massively abundant constituent of the infected cell; for example E4 polypeptides comprise up to 30 per cent of the protein mass of HPV1-induced skin warts (Doorbar *et al.* 1986). In accord with this abundance of E4 polypeptides, the most plentiful mRNA in such warts is the spliced E1^E4 species (Palermo-Dilts *et al.* 1990) which encodes a protein doublet of 16Kd and 17kD. The former consists of the whole E1^E4 fusion containing five E1 amino acids whereas the latter lacks those five, presumably via proteolytic cleavage. In addition to these species several other, higher molecular weight, E4-related species have been identified. Some are dimeric forms of the 16 and 17 kD polypeptides but others appear to be more complex and are of indeterminate structure (Doorbar *et al.* 1988). Their intracellular location is primarily cytoplasmic (Sterling *et al.* 1993).

In spite of the plentiful abundance of E4 within some infected cells the function(s) of these proteins are still something of a mystery. However, in cultured epithelial cells the E4 proteins have been shown to associate with cytokeratins, leading to the collapse of the intermediate filament network within the cell. It has been suggested that this may enhance virus release from the productively infected cell (Doorbar *et al.* 1991). On the other hand, such a dramatic cytoskeletal collapse was not observed in a different culture system where the epithelial cells remained stratified (Sterling *et al.* 1993). It remains a possibility that interactions between E4 and cytokeratins may be of importance in determining the tissue specificity of different types of HPV.

2.4.4   E5

The E5 ORF has, until relatively recently, been studied mainly in BPV. In this virus the ORF is expressed as a small polypeptide, a mere 44 amino acids in length. Much of the interest in this gene product stems from the fact that it can transform cells in culture and appears to play a major role in cellular transformation by the whole virus (reviewed by DiMaio and Neary, 1990). A potential mechanism for E5-mediated transformation is suggested by the finding that expression of E5 activates the endogenous cellular receptor for platelet-derived growth factor (PDGFR) by forming a stable complex between E5 and the receptor. This could then transmit the transforming proliferative signal to the cell (Petti *et al.* 1991; Petti and DiMaio, 1992). An additional interaction of E5 is with the 16k integral membrane subunit of the vacuolar ATPase and this association seems to be required for maximum transformation efficiency (Goldstein *et al.* 1992a). The three proteins E5, PDGFR, and 16k appear to interact together in a large complex (Goldstein *et al.* 1992b).

In the HPV system it is clear that the products of the E6 and E7 ORFs are the major transforming proteins (see Chapter 5). However, the earlier BPV work (Martin *et al.* 1989), which showed that E5 could cooperate with other growth factor receptors such as EGF and CSF-1 to induce transformation, stimulated the search for analogous interactions in HPV 16. HPV16 E5 alone was demonstrated to transform murine keratinocytes but not fibroblasts (BPV1 E5 transforms both cell types) (Leptak *et al.* 1991) and this transforming capacity was enhanced in the presence of EGF but not PDGF. E5 expressing cells were also augmented in their capacity for signal transduction to the nucleus as assayed by the level of c-fos mRNA (Leechanachai *et al.* 1992). It is currently unclear as to whether or not HPV E5 contributes to the development of human tumours. It certainly does not appear to be required for the progression and maintenance of HPV-associated lesions since the ORF is often deleted following integration of the virus genome into the host chromosomal DNA. However, in view of the E5 transforming potential *in vitro*, it is conceivable that this polypeptide may play a role in the initiation of the malignant process during the early stages prior to episomal integration.

2.4.5 L1

The L1 ORF encodes the major capsid protein of mature papillomavirus virions. The virus particle consists of an icosahedral array (Crawford and Crawford, 1963) of major (L1) and minor (L2) capsid proteins. The structure is similar to that of the polyomaviruses (Baker *et al.* 1989) and is formed from 72 pentameric capsomeres each composed of five L1 molecules and having T = 7 symmetry (Baker *et al.* 1991). Recently, several laboratories have shown that L1 proteins from a variety of HPV types, following expression in various recombinant systems, will self-assemble to produce virus-like particles (Hagensee *et al.* 1993, Rose *et al.* 1993, Kirnbauer *et al.* 1993).

The L1 polypeptide of HPV16 contains 4 potential N-linked glycosylation sites. Studies of the protein expressed from a recombinant vaccinia virus revealed that a minority of the product appeared to be glycosylated with high-mannose carbohydrate. However, whereas the majority of the L1 was non-glycosylated and localized in the nucleus, the glycosylated form seemed to be trapped in the endoplasmic reticulum. These observations suggest that the glycosylated form of L1 is unlikely to be an important part of the virion (Zhou *et al.* 1993).

Early work on serological responses to disrupted virions or denatured L1 protein pointed to there being antibody cross-reactivity between different papillomavirus types, suggesting that L1 might be the papillomavirus 'group-specific antigen' (Jenson *et al.* 1980; Doorbar and Gallimore 1987; Banks *et al.* 1987). In systems that can support an assay for infection by the virus (e.g. BPV) it was found that such antisera would not neutralize virus infectivity. However, like intact BPV virions, the virus-like particles generated in self-assembly experiments were found to be highly immunogenic and induced neutralizing antibodies. Thus it seems that such neutralizing antibodies recognize conformational rather than linear epitopes. Recent data also point to the possibility of type specific conformational epitopes of L1.

Virus neutralization by L1 antibodies has obvious implications for vaccine development to combat HPV-associated diseases including cervical carcinoma. This topic is addressed in Chapter 10.

2.4.6 L2

As mentioned above the product of the L2 ORF is the second, minor component of the virus capsid. The precise localization of L2 protein within the virion is still not clear. However, self-assembly experiments suggest a higher degree of heterogeneity in virus-like particles containing L1 alone when compared to those consisting of both L1 and L2. This implies a role for L2 in the stabilization of the capsid structure (Hagensee *et al.* 1993).

L2 has shown some promise as the basis for potential HPV diagnostic tests since, at least for HPVs 16 and 18, naturally occuring antisera are frequently directed against this protein and are mostly type-specific (Jenison *et al.* 1991; Komly *et al.* 1986). These results are being refined with a view to producing high titre, type-specific peptide antisera for use as immunological probes (Volpers *et al.* 1993).

2.5   Intratypic variation

It would be imagined that a huge, worldwide pool of replicating and evolving organisms would show sequence divergence to a greater or lesser degree depending on selective constraints. Some investigations have been performed which begin to address the question of genetic variability within, rather than between, HPV types. Ter Meulen *et al.* (1993) examined the E7 ORF from 26 isolates of HPV18 DNA and found 6 different mutations, 4 of which resulted in amino acid changes. Chan *et al.* (1992a) examined the LCR and E5 coding region from 118 HPV16 isolates. They detected 42 points of mutation in the 364 bp enhancer region and 21 different mutation sites within E5 (252 bp). In all these cases the mutations have been single base changes which were often silent in terms of amino acid coding potential. Thus the current type designations appear to be maintained reasonably tightly.

2.5.1   Subtypes

Isolates of papillomaviruses from different sources or localities have in some cases revealed variant genomes which are closely related to a previously defined type. These different isolates are referred to as subtypes and often differ by virtue of small deletions or insertions within an otherwise well-conserved genome. For example, the prototype HPV5 genome was isolated from a wart of an epidermodysplasia verruciformis (EV) patient (Zachow *et al.* 1987). A related genome, designated HPV5b, was later isolated from a carcinoma in an EV patient. Sequence analysis of this genome and comparison with the prototype HPV5 revealed amino acid divergences of between 1.8 per cent and 6.0 per cent in the various ORFs and separation of the early and late regions of HPV5b by 39 nucleotides of noncoding sequence (Yabe *et al.* 1991). The HPV5b sequence contains an additional potential ORF (L3) within the late region. Although not present in HPV5a or any other HPV, an analogous ORF has been found in deer papillomavirus (Groff and Lancaster, 1985) and BPV4 (Patel *et al.* 1987).

2.6   Evolutionary relationships

The *Papovaviridae*, by virtue of their small genomes, are attractive subjects for DNA sequence analysis and certain members (SV40 and Polyoma) were the first DNA genomes to have their complete primary structures determined. It was not long until this opportunity for phylogenetic analysis was recognized, the results of which suggested that Polyoma virus, BK virus, and SV40 evolved from a common ancestor and diverged with their respective host species (Soeda *et al.* 1980). More recently, a study of geographical variants of HPV 16 suggested that it similarly co-evolved with humans (Chan *et al.* 1992a). A much wider study of evolutionary relationships between the sequences of papillomaviruses (infecting all species) (Chan *et al.* 1992b) reveals a complicated picture of interrelationships with evidence for virus–host co-evolution, and evolution along lines of pathology and tissue specificity. The conclusion is that the extant papillomavirus types are consistent with belonging to natural biological taxonomic units but that in view of the broad diversity of types it is not clear why there do not seem to be any 'intermediate' types. In the realms of evolutionary molecular genetics of papillomaviruses much clearly remains to be elucidated.

References

Baker, T. S., Drak, J., and Bina, M. (1989). The capsid of small papovaviruses contains 72 pentameric capsomeres: direct evidence from cryoelectron microscopy of simian virus 40. *Biophysics Journal*, **55**, 243–53.

Baker, T. S., Newcomb, W. W., Olson, N. H., Cowsert, L. M., Olson, C., and Brown, J. C. (1991). Structures of bovine and human papillomaviruses. Analysis by cryoelectron microscopy and three-dimensional image reconstruction. *Biophysical Journal*, **60**, 1445–56.

Banks, L., Matlashewski, G., Pim, D., Churcher, M., Roberts, C., and Crawford, L. V. (1987). Expression of human papillomavirus type 6 and type 16 capsid proteins in bacteria and their antigenic characterization. *Journal of General Virology*, **68**, 3081–89.

Bream, G. L., Ohmstede, C.-A., and Phelps, W. C. (1993). Characterization of human papillomavirus type 11 E1 and E2 proteins expressed in insect cells. *Journal of Virology*, **67**, 2655–63.

Chan, S.-Y., Ho, L., Ong, C.-K., Chow, V., Drescher, M., Durst, J., tet Meulen, J., Villa, L., Luande, J., Mgaya, H. N., and Bernard, H. U. (1992a). Molecular variants of human papillomavirus-16 from four continents suggest pandemic spread of the virus and its coevolution with humankind. *Journal of Virology*, **66**, 2057–66.

Chan, S.-Y., Bernard, H.-U., Ong, C.-K., Chan, S.-P., Hoffman, B., and Delius, H. (1992b). Phylogenetic analysis of 48 papillomavirus types and 28 subtypes and variants: a showcase for the molecular evolution of DNA viruses. *Journal of Virology*, **66**, 5714–25.

Chiang, C.-M., Broker, T. M., and Chow, L. T. (1991). An E1M^E2C fusion protein encoded by human papillomavirus type 11 is a sequence-specific transcription repressor. *Journal of Virology*, **65**, 3317–29.

Crawford, L. V. and Crawford, E. M. (1963). A comparative study of polyoma and papillomavirus. *Virology*, **21**, 258–63.

DiMaio, D. and Neary, K. (1990). The genetics of bovine papillomavirus type 1. In *Papillomaviruses and human cancer* (ed. H. Pfister), pp. 113–44. CRC Press, Boca Raton.

Doorbar, J., Campbell, D., Grand, R. J. A., and Gallimore, P. H. (1986). Identification of the human papillomavirus-1a gene products. *EMBO Journal*, **5**, 355–62.

Doorbar, J., Evans, H. S., Coneron, I., Crawford, L. V., and Gallimore, P. H. (1988). Analysis of HPV-1 E4 gene expression using epitope-defined antibodies. *EMBO Journal*, **7**, 825–33.

Doorbar, J. and Gallimore, P. H. (1987). Identification of proteins encoded by the L1 and L2 open reading frames of human papillomavirus 1a. *Journal of Virology*, **61**, 2793–99.

Doorbar, J., Parton, A., Hartley, K., Banks, L., Crook, T., Stanley, M., and Crawford, L. (1990). Detection of novel splicing patterns in a HPV 16-containing keratinocyte cell line. *Virology*, **178**, 254–62.

Doorbar, J, Ely, S., Sterling, J., McLean, C., and Crawford, L. (1991). Specific interaction between HPV-16 E1-E4 and cytokeratins results in collapse of the epithelial cell intermediate filament network. *Nature*, **352**, 824–27.

Goldstein, D. J., Kulke, R., DiMaio, D., and Schlegel, R. (1992a). A glutamine residue in the membrane-associating domain of the bovine papillomavirus type 1 E5 oncoprotein mediates its binding to a transmembrane component of the vacuolar H+-ATPase. *Journal of Virology*, **66**, 405–13.

Goldstein, D. J., Andresson, T., Sparkowski, J. J., and Schlegel, R. (1992b). The BPV-1 E5 protein, the 16kDa membrane pore-forming protein and the PDGF receptor exist in a complex that is dependent on hydrophobic transmembrane interactions. *EMBO Journal*, **11**, 4851–59.

Green, M., Mackey, J. K., Wold, W. S., and Rigden, P. (1979). Thirty one human Adenovirus serotypes (Ad1-Ad31) form five groups (A-E) based upon DNA genome homologies. *Virology*, **93**, 481–92.

Groff, D. A. and Lancaster, W. D. (1985). Molecular cloning and nucleotide sequence of deer papillomavirus. *Journal of Virology*, **56**, 85–91.

Hagensee, M. E., Yaegashi, N., and Galloway, D. A. (1993). Self-assembly of human papillomavirus type 1 capsids by expression of the L1 protein alone or by coexpression of the L1 and L2 capsid proteins. *Journal of Virology*, **67**, 315–22.

Hermonat, P. L. and Howley, P. M. (1987). Mutational analysis of the 3' open reading frames and the splice junction at nucleotide 3225 of bovine papillomavirus type 1. *Journal of Virology*, **61**, 3889–95.

Jackson, R., Howell, M. T., and Kaminski (1990). The novel mechanism of initiation of picornavirus RNA translation. *Trends in Biochemical Science*, **15**, 477–83.

Jenison, S. A., Yu, X.-P., Valentine, J. M., and Galloway, D. A. (1991). Characterization of human antibody-reactive epitopes encoded by human papillomavirus types 16 and 18. *Journal of Virology*, **65**, 1208–18.

Jenson, A. B., Rosenthal, J. D., Olson, C., Pass, F., Lancaster, W. D., and Shah, K. (1980). Immunological relatedness of papillomaviruses from different species. *Journal of the National Cancer Institute*, **64**, 495–500.

Kirnbauer, R., Booy, F., Cheng, N., Lowy, D. R., and Schiller, J. T. (1992). Papillomavirus L1 major capsid protein self-assembles into virus-like particles that are highly immunogenic. *Proceedings of the National Academy of Sciences U.S.A.*, **89**, 12180–84.

Komly, C. A., Breitburd, F., Croissant, O., and Streek, R. E. (1986). The L2 open reading frame of human papillomavirus type 1a encodes a minor structural protein carrying type-specific antigens. *Journal of Virology*, **60**, 813–16.

Kozak, M. (1987) An analysis of 5′ noncoding sequences from 699 vertebrate messenger RNAs. *Nucleic Acids Research*, **15**, 8125–48.

Kozak, M. (1989). The scanning model for translation: an update. *Journal of Cell Biology*, **108**, 229–41.

Leechanachai, P., Banks, L., Moreau, F., and Matlashewski, G. (1992). The E5 gene from human papillomavirus type 16 is an oncogene which enhances growth factor-mediated signal transduction to the nucleus. *Oncogene*, **7**, 19–25.

Leptak, C., Ramon y Cajal, S., Kulke, R., Horwitz, B. H., Riese, D. J. II, Dotto, G. P., and DiMaio, D. (1991). Tumorigenic transformation of murine keratinocytes by the E5 genes of bovine papillomavirus type 1 and human papillomavirus type 16. *Journal of Virology*, **65**, 7078–83.

Martin, P., Vass, W. C., Schiller, J. T., Lowy, D. R., and Velu, T. J. (1989). The bovine papillomavirus-E5 transforming protein can stimulate the transforming activity of EGF and CSF-1 receptors. *Cell*, **59**, 21–32.

Münger, K., Phelps, W. C., Bubb, V., Howley, P. M., and Schlegel, R. (1989). The E6 and E7 genes of the human papillomavirus type 16 together are necessary and sufficient for transformation of primary human Keratinocytes. *Journal of Virology*, **63**, 4417–21.

Palermo-Dilts, D. A., Broker, T. R., and Chow, L. T. (1990). Human papillomavirus type 1 produces redundant as well as polycistronic mRNAs in plantar warts. *Journal of Virology*, **64**, 3144–9.

Patel, K. R., Smith, K. T., and Campo, M. S. (1987). The nucleotide sequence and genome organization of bovine papillomavirus type 4. *Journal of General Virology*, **68**, 2117–28.

Petti, L. and DiMaio, D. (1992). Stable association between the bovine papillomavirus E5 transforming protein and activated platelet-derived growth factor receptor in transformed mouse cells. *Proceedings of the National Academy Sciences U.S.A.*, **89**, 6736–40.

Petti, L., Nilson, L. A., and Di Maio, D. (1991). Activation of the platelet-derived growth factor receptor by the bovine papillomavirus E5 transforming protein. *EMBO Journal*, **10**, 845–55.

Rohlfs, M., Winkenbach, S., Meyer, S., Rupp, T., and Dürst, M. (1991). Viral transcription in human keratinocyte cell line immortalized by human papillomavirus type-16. *Virology*, **183**, 331–42.

Romanczuk, H. and Howley, P. M. (1992) Disruption of either the E1 or the E2 regulatory gene of human papillomavirus type 16 increases viral immortalization capacity. *Proceedings of the National Academy Sciences U.S.A.*, **89**, 3159–63.

Rose, R. C., Bonnez, W., Reichman, R. C., and Garcea, R. L. (1993). Expression of human papillomavirus type 11 L1 protein in insect cells: *In vivo* and *in vitro* assembly of viruslike particles. *Journal of Virology*, **67**, 1936–44.

Sherman, L., Alloul, N., Golan, I., Dürst, M., and Baram, A. (1992). Expression and splicing patterns of human papillomavirus type-16 mRNAs in precancerous lesions and carcinoma of the cervix, in human keratinocytes immortalized by HPV 16, and in cell lines established from cervical cancers. *International Journal of Cancer*, **50**, 356–64.

Smotkin, D., Prokoph, H., and Wettstein, F. E. (1989). Oncogenic and nononcogenic human genital papillomaviruses generate the E7 mRNA by different mechanisms. *Journal of Virology*, **63**, 1441–47.

Soeda, E., Maruyama, T., Arrand, J. R., and Griffin, B. E. (1980). Host-dependent evolution of three papova viruses. *Nature*, **285**, 165–67.

Sterling, J. C., Stanley, M. A., Gatward, G., and Minson, A. C. (1990). Production of HPV 16 virions by a human keratinocyte cell line. *Journal of Virology*, **64**, 6305–07.

Sterling, J. C., Skepper, J. N., and Stanley, M. A. (1993). Immunoelectron microscopical localization of human papillomavirus type 16 L1 and E4 proteins in cervical keratinocytes cultured *in vivo*. *Journal of Investigative Dermatology*, **100**, 154–58.

Storey, A., Greenfield, I., Banks, L. Pim, D., Crook, T., Crawford, L., and Stanley, M. (1992). Lack of immortalizing activity of a human papillomavirus type 16 variant DNA with a mutation in the E2 gene isolated from normal human cervical keratinocytes. *Oncogene*, **7**, 459–65.

Volpers, C., Sapp, M., Komly, C. A., Richalet-Secordel, P., and Streek, R. E. (1993). Development of type-specific and cross-reactive serological probes for the minor capsid protein of human papillomavirus type 33. *Journal of Virology*, **67**, 1927–35.

Wang, F., Petti, L., Braun, D., Seung, S., and Kieff, E. (1987). A bicistronic Epstein–Barr virus mRNA encodes two nuclear proteins in latently infected, growth-transformed lymphocytes. *Journal of Virology*, **61**, 945–54.

Yabe,Y., Sakai, A., Hitsumoto, T., Kato, H., and Ogura, H. (1991). A subtype of human papillomavirus 5 (HPV5b) and its subgenomic segment amplified in a carcinoma: nucleotide sequences and genomic organizations. *Virology*, **183**, 793–8.

Yang, L., Mohr, I., Fouts, E., Lim, D. A., Nohaile, M., and Botchan, M. (1993). The E1 protein of bovine papillomavirus 1 is an ATP-dependent DNA helicase. *Proceedings of the National Academy Sciences. U.S.A.*, **90**, 5086–90.

Zachow, K. R., Ostrow, R. S., and Faras, A. J. (1987). Nucleotide-sequence and genome organization of human papillomavirus type 5. *Virology*, **158**, 251–4.

Zhou, J., Sun, X.-Y., Stenzel, D. J., and Frazer, I. H. (1991). Expression of vaccinia recombinant HPV16 L1 and L2 ORF proteins in epithelial cells is sufficient for assembly of HPV virion-like particles. *Virology*, **185**, 251–7.

Zhou, J., Sun, X.-Y., and Frazer, I. H. (1993). Glycosylation of human papillomavirus type 16 L1 protein. *Virology*, **194**, 210–18.

3 Detection of genital human papillomavirus infections: Critical review of methods and prevalence studies in relation to cervical cancer

JAN M. M. WALBOOMERS, ANA-MARIA
DE RODA HUSMAN, ADRIAAN J. C. VAN
DEN BRULE, PETER J. F. SNIJDERS, and
CHRIS J. L. M. MEIJER

3.1 Introduction and historical perspectives

More than a century ago sexual activity was already considered as an important risk factor for the development of cancer of the uterine cervix (cervical cancer). As early as 1842 Regioni-Stern described that this type of cancer rarely exists in nuns and is frequently observed in prostitutes. Other epidemiological studies have shown that onset of sexual activity at an early age and promiscuity are important risk factors for this disease (Rotkin 1967). In addition it was noted that in monogamous women cervical cancer was more frequently detected if the male partner had penile cancer, more sexual partners, or had already been previously married to a woman who died from cervical cancer. All these observations point to the involvement of an infectious agent in the etiology of human genital cancer. Candidate micro-organisms which have been critically studied include bacteria (*Treponema pallidum*, *Neisseria gonorrhoe*, *Chlamydia trachomatis*), protozoa (*Trichomonas vaginalis*), and viruses (herpes simplex virus and cytomegalo virus) but these appear to be of minor importance. Since 1970 the possible involvement of human papillomavirus infections in the etiology of human genital cancer has been under investigation (Zur Hausen 1977, 1989, 1991; Gissmann and Schneider 1986). Originally a single human papillomavirus was believed only to cause benign skin warts, papillomas, and warts on the genitals (condylomas). Electron microscopy identified small viral particles of the same size (45–50 nm in diameter) in both skin warts and condylomata and these were characterized as small DNA viruses of the family *papovaviridae*. Transmission experiments using extracts of skin warts or condylomata proved to induce warts in volunteers. Further HPV research was hampered by the difficulty of *in vitro* virus production because of the latter's dependence on the differentiation of the squamous epithelium *in vivo*.

In 1976 Zur Hausen pointed out that genital warts show an identical epidemiological pattern as cervical cancer and postulated that a papillomavirus could be involved in the development of cervical cancer. Moreover, cytologists frequently reported the presence of HPV-induced cellular abnormalities called koilocytes in cytological smears of women with mainly mild morphological changes while condylomas could not be detected (Meisels and Morin 1981).

In the early 1980s Zur Hausen and Gissmann made an important breakthrough in human papillomavirus research by isolating and characterizing HPV DNA from condylomata and laryngeal papillomas by molecular cloning. This HPV DNA demonstrated less than 50 per cent homology by liquid hybridization with other HPVs isolated from skin warts; this criterion formed the basis for the classification of new HPV types.

In initial epidemiological studies it was believed that there were only two benign or low-risk HPV types (HPV 6 and 11) and two oncogenic or high-risk HPV types (HPV 16 and 18). Thus HPV 6 and 11 were mainly found in benign cervical lesions while HPV 16 and 18 were mainly present in pre-malignant and malignant cervical lesions. This was substantiated in an early follow-up study of 100 women with mild dysplastic cervical lesions (CIN I) of which 26 developed a carcinoma *in situ* (CIN III) over a period of about 30 months. Of these women 22 (85 per cent) were HPV 16 positive. Regression was mainly found in HPV 16 negative lesions (Campion *et al.* 1986).

Subsequently, the number of HPV genotypes identified has increased dramatically and the plurality of these viruses has became clear. To date more than 70 different HPV genotypes have been isolated from different lesions found in mucosal epithelium and skin (De Villiers 1989). In Table 3.1 only the mucosotropic HPV genotypes affecting the anogenital and oral region are listed.

The degree of DNA homology between different HPV types varies considerably. For example, HPV 6, 11, and 13 are very similar while HPV 41 shows almost no homology with other known types. It has recently been proposed that the classification of HPVs be based on less than 90 per cent sequence homology in the ORFs E6, E7, and L1 to any other known HPV type.

HPV detection by nucleic acid hybridization is currently the best diagnostic tool available. Thus while viral infections can often be diagnosed by virus culture, this is not possible for HPV. Detection of HPV particles in genital lesions using transmission electron microscopy is not practical for screening purposes. Immunohistochemical detection of HPV antigens has

Table 3.1 Overview of mucosotropic HPV genotypes

HPV genotype	Associated with[1]
6	condyloma acuminata, CIN
11	laryngeal papilloma, CIN
13	focal epithelial hyperplasia
16	CIN, cervical carcinoma
18	CIN, cervical carcinoma
30	CIN, laryngeal carcinoma
31	CIN, cervical carcinoma
32	focal epithelial hyperplasia, oral papilloma
33	CIN, cervical carcinoma
34	CIN
35	CIN, cervical carcinoma
39	CIN, cervical carcinoma, PIN
40	CIN, PIN
42	CIN, vulvar papilloma
43	CIN, vulvar hyperplasia
44	CIN, vulvar condyloma
45	CIN, cervical carcinoma
51	CIN, cervical carcinoma
52	CIN, cervical carcinoma
53	normal cervical mucosa
54	condyloma acuminata
55	Bowenoid papulosis
56	CIN, cervical carcinoma
57	CIN, inverted papilloma
58	CIN
59	VIN

[1] PIN, VIN, CIN: penile, vulvar, and cervical intra-epithelial neoplasia respectively

(Modified from De Villiers 1989).

been shown using antisera directed against capsid proteins of BPV (cross reactive with all PV types including HPV). However, this approach probably only identifies productive HPV infections associated with condylomas and mild dysplastic lesions and which are absent in invasive cancer. The detection by immunohistochemistry of HPV early protein expression in cervical lesions using specific antibodies or of patient serological responses to HPV antigens are currently being evaluated but cannot substitute for HPV nucleic detection.

Genome organization of HPVs (see Chapter 2, Fig. 2.1) has been defined by analogy to bovine papillomavirus type 1 (BPV 1). All HPV genotypes with determined nucleotide sequence showed similar genome organization.

Homology comparisons between these types reveal the strongest conservation in the E1 and L1 ORFs. These conserved regions can contribute in a high degree to cross-hybridization in the detection of a particular HPV type. On the other hand, this characteristic is of important value in HPV detection as described later.

All available techniques for detection of HPV specific nucleic acids share the basic principle of hybridization: pairing of complementary single-stranded DNA (RNA) strands resulting in the formation of double-stranded hybrids. This means that HPV DNA (RNA) present in a sample is detected on the basis of its ability to hybridize with a probe. Purified HPV DNA (RNA) provided with a (non-) radioactive label serves as probe. Labelled hybrids are visualized by autoradiography (exposure to an X-ray-sensitive film) or immunohistochemical staining procedures. Efficiency of hybridization is dependent on:

(1) the extent of homology in nucleotide sequences between probe and target DNA;

(2) reaction conditions including ionic strength of hybridization solution and temperature.

By varying these conditions, it is possible to change the stringency of hybridization. High-stringent hybridization enables only complete homologous DNAs to form hybrids, while under low-stringent conditions heterologous or less homologous DNA also hybridize.

HPV nucleic acid detection has been revolutionized during the last years. In the following section an inventory and critical review of the most frequently applied methods will be given. Emphasis will be placed on the the recently introduced polymerase chain reaction method (Mullis and Faloona 1987; Ehrlich *et al.* 1991).

3.2   Detection of genital HPV infections

3.2.1   Clinical detection of HPV infections

The spectrum of genital HPV infections are divided into latent, subclinical, clinical, and HPV-associated neoplasia. Clinical HPV infections are visible with the naked eye and may cause symptoms to the patient. Subclinical HPV infections do not cause symptoms but produce subtle flat lesions which can only be diagnosed after acetic acid treatment by colposcope. The morphological abnormalities can be substantiated by light microscopy. In contrast, latent HPV infections cannot be diagnosed by colposcopy, cytology, or histology since the presence of the virus does not cause any morphological abnormalities in the infected tissue. HPV infections are differentiated from HPV-associated neoplasia because it seems that other factors in addition to HPV are needed to induce malignant transformation of the genital squamous epithelium.

Although the detection of HPV infections using colposcopy, histology, and cytology has been claimed, these techniques are not able to identify the virus itself, but detect the (sub-) clinical manifestation of the HPV infection. Moreover, the formation of koilocytes, the main cytological and histological criterion for HPV infection, and 'HPV-specific' colposcopic pattern, can also be caused by agents other than HPV. In addition, koilocytes can be absent in HPV infections. Thus the sensitivity and specificity of these techniques in HPV detection are low and rather controversial. Furthermore, they fail to discriminate between the different types of HPV.

3.2.2   Molecular biological detection of HPV infections

Two types of HPV DNA detection methods are frequently applied based on either direct detection of HPV DNA or HPV-DNA amplification.

3.2.3   HPV detection without DNA amplification

Southern blot (SB) analysis

Purified target DNA, either digested with specific restriction enzymes or uncut, is electrophoretically separated on the basis of size of DNA fragments. DNA is subsequently transferred to a DNA binding filter support and hybridized with HPV type specific probes. Since each HPV type has a specific fragmentation pattern after restriction enzyme digestion, the HPV hybridization signals can be interpreted by comparison to standard hybridization patterns of HPV prototypes. Therefore both the probe used and the resulting hybridization pattern are valuable markers which together determine the outcome of the typing. By varying the hybridization conditions (lower stringency) heterologous DNA fragments can also be detected, identifying still undefined HPV types (HPV-X). An additional advantage of the Southern blot technique is that it can provide information about the physical state of HPV in the sample investigated. As shown in Fig. 3.1, Southern blot analysis can distinguish between episomal (Fig. 3.1A,C) and integrated viral DNA (Fig. 3.1B,D), which might be of importance for the transition of pre-malignant lesions to cervical cancer. Episomal DNA is mainly found in benign lesions while integrated HPV DNA is mainly detected in cervical cancer. Moreover, sometimes rearrangements in the genome can also be detected (Fig. 3.1C).

SB analysis is considered to be the 'golden standard' for HPV detection and typing. Although SB analysis is sensitive (about 1 pg HPV DNA in 10 μg genomic DNA can be detected) and specific, the technique is laborious and requires large quantities of DNA (5-10 μg) which is relevant for small tissue samples like biopsies. Recently, Brandsma *et al.* (1989) described

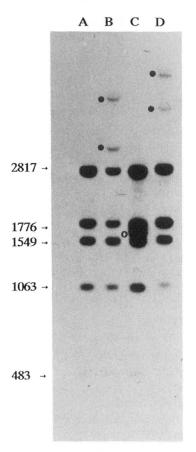

Fig. 3.1 Southern blot analysis of HPV 16 positive cervical carcinoma. A normal Pst1 pattern of HPV 16 DNA resulting in 2818, 1776, 1549, 1063, and 1483 base pair fragments is visible in all lanes. In lanes B and D additional bands (dotted circles) are visible indicating integration of the HPV 16 genome into chromosomal DNA. In lane C DNA fragment indicated by open circle appeared to be part of URR showing genome rearrangement.

the results of a comparative study in different laboratories with extensive experience using SB analysis for HPV detection and typing. Interlaboratory HPV detection agreements ranged from 66 to 97 per cent while interlaboratory HPV typing agreement ranged from 77 to 96 per cent. When differences regarding HPV presence and typing were combined the results were in agreement for all laboratories for only 45 per cent of the samples. It is clearly questionable whether this technique is sufficiently reliable for use as a golden standard.

Dot blot analysis/ViraPap

This method differs from SB analysis in that the DNA is fixed onto the membrane and is not electrophoretically separated. Relatively small quantities of DNA (0.3–1.0 μg) are required and sensitivities of about 0.5–1 pg HPV DNA in 1 μg genomic DNA can be achieved. There are two variants: one uses DNA probes (dot blot), the other uses RNA probes (ViraPap).

Concerning the DNA/DNA situation the procedure can only be performed reliably under high-stringency conditions and even then it is difficult to differentiate between related HPV types.

The most commonly used dot blot assay is the ViraPap/ViraType system, the only HPV test currently approved by the Food and Drug Administration for clinical use in the USA. The assay system contains RNA probes to detect HPV DNA presence (ViraPap) and type (ViraType) for a limited number of HPV types: 6, 11, 16, 18, 31, 33, and 35. The system can only be appropriately compared with other techniques for the seven types included in the test. Initially the system was based on radioactive probes but recently a non-radioisotopic detection system with possibilities for quantitation has been introduced.

Filter in situ *hybridization (FISH)*

In contrast to Southern blot and dot blot techniques, extraction of DNA is not required for the filter *in situ* hybridization (FISH) technique (Wagner *et al.* 1984). Cervical scrapes are spotted directly onto a membrane where the DNA is denatured. HPV positive samples can be identified by hybridization with HPV-specific probes. Despite modifications to the FISH the method lacks sensitivity. The sensitivity of the FISH was estimated to be at best half the sensitivity of the Southern blot technique. Besides this the FISH is hampered by high background signals. More importantly, no association was found between HPV infection and known risk factors for cervical neoplasia, while strong associations have been observed using other methods.

In situ *hybridization (ISH)*

The strength of the *in situ* hybridization technique is the preservation of morphology of the specimen which permits localization of HPV within the tissue and the infected cell (Brigati *et al.* 1983). Pre-treatment of tissue consisting of partial digestion of cellular and nuclear proteins is necessary for target DNA to become accessible to the probe. The DNA *in situ* hybridization technique has a sensitivity of 20–50 HPV genomes per cell, in particular when full genomic length, non-radioactive labelled probes are used (Brigati *et al.* 1983). The requirement of biopsies makes this method unsuitable for mass screening but the possibility of determining the localization of the viral genome and analysing its expression pattern (RNA *in situ* hybridization) is of great value in research on the pathogenesis of cervical cancer (Stoler *et al.* 1990). The definition of subclinical and latent HPV infection is still incomplete and awaits clarification by highly sensitive HPV detection systems that preserve the morphology of the tissue. Thus far, the application of *in situ* hybridization to morphologically normal epithelium suspected to be latently infected has detected no viral DNA (Syranen and Syranen 1989).

3.2.4   Detection of HPV DNA after amplification by polymerase chain reaction

Principle of polymerase chain reaction

The polymerase chain reaction (PCR) is an enzymatic *in vitro* amplification of a piece of 'target' DNA. The technique is based on the annealing of two short oligonucleotides (primers) of about 20 nucleotides to the opposite strands of a certain denatured target DNA molecule (i.e. small part of the HPV genome), thereby providing free $3'$-OH ends for DNA polymerase mediated chain primer elongation. Primers are chosen in a way that they flank a piece of 50–500 bases. Thus the process includes three steps: (a) denaturation of target DNA (94 °C, 1 min); (b) primer annealing (37–70 °C); and (c) primer elongation (72 °C), generating daughter strands of DNA that encompass the region between the two primers. Usually 30–40 cycles of amplification are performed, achieving an exponential increase in the amount of target DNA spanned by both primers. In Fig. 3.2 the principle of the PCR is schematically illustrated.

Under optimal conditions a two-fold increase in the amount of target DNA can be obtained during each cycle. Theoretically a million-fold increase of the amplification product can be obtained after performance of twenty PCR cycles (2^{20} = 1 048 576). Therefore a sensitivity of 1 HPV copy per sample can be reached by PCR. Ultimately, amplified DNA often can be resolved at the agarose gel level but additional hybridization by dot- or Southern blotting using target DNA specific probes originating from the internal part of the amplified DNA is necessary to confirm specificity. In addition, sensitivity is at least ten times increased by this hybridization step. Radioactive and non-radioactive probes have been used successfully. PCR products can also be analysed by digestion with restriction enzymes. Some primer sets for HPV detection generate amplification products that contain unique restriction enzymes digestion patterns that can be used for HPV typing. Also the identification of novel HPV types is possible using this approach.

Advantages and disadvantages of PCR

The PCR method is not only advantageous because of its high sensitivity and specificity but also by its requirement of relatively low amounts of

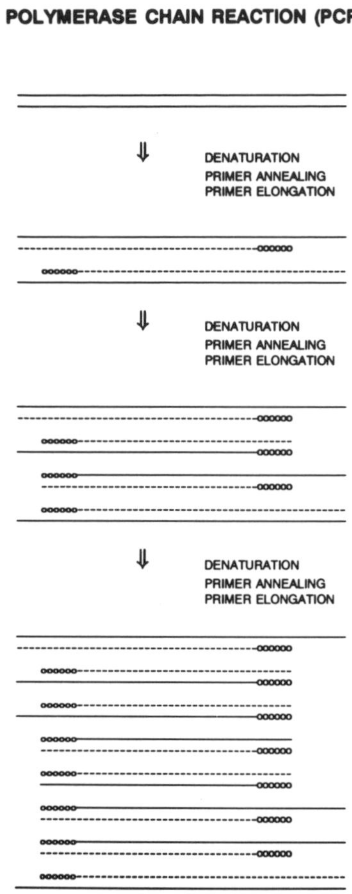

POLYMERASE CHAIN REACTION (PCR)

Fig. 3.2   Principle of PCR. For explanation see text.

target DNA (25 to 500 ng) which is important in the case of small tissue specimens. Another advantage is that the PCR can be applied to crude cell suspensions, that is, cervical smears, and formalin fixed paraffin embedded tissue. The application to crude cervical scrapes is the most important prerequisite to the use of PCR for large screening programmes by circumventing the laborious and time-consuming DNA extraction procedures and minimizing sample-to-sample contamination. It appeared that non-ionic detergent/protease K digestion and even freezing, thawing, and boiling of cell suspension is sufficient for successful amplification of HPV target sequences (Van den Brule *et al.* 1990a).

Ironically the major drawback of the PCR method is its sensitivity that is, its susceptibility to contamination. Minute amounts of recombinant

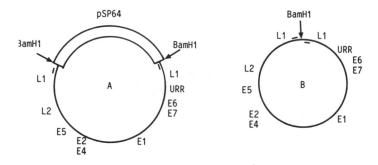

Fig. 3.3 Principle of anticontamination primers. Bars indicate primers flanking the BamH1 cloning site and (A) direct the amplification of the 3 kbp SP64 fragment, or (B) direct the amplification of a 200 bp fragment of episomal HPV DNA. The PCR conditions used are optimal for the amplification of up to a 500 bp fragment. E = early genes; L = late genes; URR = regulatory region.

plasmids and PCR products can give rise to false positive results. Several early reports that used PCR-based methods to detect HPV were unreliable because of such problems and some have since been retracted. In order to avoid false positives from plasmid HPVs (pHPV), the use of anticontamination primers or cloning site flanking primers was introduced (see Fig. 3.3). Application of these primers makes it possible to detect HPVs specifically in a clinical sample even in the presence of pHPVs (Van den Brule *et al.* 1989). However, amplification products are the most serious source of contamination and therefore it is necessary to carry out the different PCR steps, such as sample preparation, electrophoresis, and PCR solution preparation in three different and separated rooms. This requires strong laboratory discipline. During the whole procedure, the use of disposable tubes and special pipette tips is also necessary. An alternative to prevent carry-over of amplification products has recently been developed, which involves the incorporation of deoxyuridinetriphosphate (dUTP) and the enzyme uracil N glycosylase (UNG)(Longo *et al.* 1992). Treatment of the PCR product by UNG at alkaline pH and elevated temperature destroys exogenous uracil containing PCR products.

With these precautions, the direct HPV-PCR is can be performed reliably.

HPV type specific primer mediated PCR

Since the PCR carried out on crude samples is easy to perform, a trained technician can routinely screen at least 500 samples a week. Initially HPV type specific PCRs have been developed and applied to a variety of clinical specimens.

Sequence data of the mucosotropic HPV types 6, 11, 16, 18, 31, and 33 were first available for primer selection. Using computer-assisted matrix

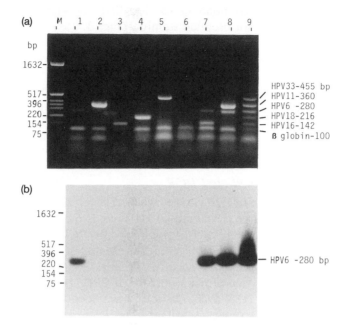

Fig. 3.4 Detection of HPV genotypes. Crude cervical scrapes were analysed using the PCR with a mixture of anticontamination primer sets specific to different HPV types. Lanes 1–5, 7, and 8 contained samples from HPV-positive patients. Lane 6 contained a sample from an HPV-negative patient. In the last lane, a mixture of the DNAs of patients 1–5 is shown. The β-globin amplification was used as an internal control. (a) PCR products are shown after electrophoresis on 2 per cent agarose gel and ethidium bromide staining; (b) Southern blot analysis with an HPV 6 specific oligonucleotide probe. M:pBR322xHinfI.

comparison analysis (Microgenic, Gen Bank, Release # 154) it is easy to design HPV type specific primers. HPV type specific primers have been developed for several parts of the HPV genomes and could be synthesized in large amounts *in vitro*. To limit the number of PCRs to be carried out a mixture of HPV type specific primers pairs can be used in one PCR reaction (multiplex PCR). For that purpose primers pairs have been selected in such a manner that for the several HPV types different amplified fragment sizes were generated. Also a β globin PCR is included which serves as an internal DNA quality control.

Based on this approach in Fig. 3.4 an example of the results of HPV type specific PCRs for HPV 6, 11, 16, 18, and 33 applied on cervical smears is shown. Also a multipex PCR for these five HPV types was performed in a mixture of different cervical smears (lane 9). In these samples the amplified bands, corresponding to the different HPV types, can be seen already after ethidium bromide staining (Fig. 3.4(a)). However, multiplex PCR is hampered by a reduced sensitivity. Therefore PCR carried out with a maximum of two pairs primers (duplex PCR) is advised for optimal HPV detection.

Figure 3.4(b) shows the results after Southern blot analysis using a HPV 6 specific probe (30 oligonucleotides) originating from the internal part of the amplified product. At present, type specific PCR assays can be extended for other types by selecting additional primers from newly available sequence data.

HPV general primer mediated PCR

Since more than 24 genital HPV types with different oncogenic potential have been isolated it will be clear that for HPV epidemiology not all samples can be screened for all these types by type specific PCR but that it is very convenient to explore the possibility of developing a test discriminating between HPV positive and HPV negative samples. Therefore primer pairs were developed to amplify a broad spectrum of HPV types.

Different generalized HPV PCR methods have been described by several groups using general or consensus primers located in the E1 and L1 HPV genes, because matrix comparison of the sequenced HPV 6, 11, 16, 18, 31, and 33 revealed that these regions were the most conserved. Since the largest nucleotide homology amongst the sequenced HPVs does not exceed 12 consecutive nucleotides, all groups have adapted either the primers or the method to ensure amplification of a broad spectrum of HPVs. Adaptations include a certain degree of mismatched acceptance between primers and target DNA accomplished by reducing the stringency of primer annealing (Snijders *et al.* 1990; Van den Brule *et al.* 1990b), the use of degenerate primers (a mixture of oligonucleotides showing nucleotide differences at several positions) to render them sufficiently complementary to HPV 6, 11, 16, 18 and 33 (Manos *et al.* 1989) and the use of primers which in addition contain inosine residues at certain ambiguous base positions (Gregoire *et al.* 1989). Table 3.2 gives an overview of HPV consensus primers that initially have been selected and are commonly used.

Both the HPV consensus PCR with the MY 09/11 primer sets described by Manos *et al.* and the general primers G 5/6 have been succesfully applied to clinical samples in several large studies.

In the MY09/MY11 system HPV detection and typing is carried out simultaneously with dot blotting of PCR products and hybridization with radioactive- or biotin-labelled probes (HPV generic and type specific oligomers). In the GP5/6 system HPV specific PCR products are detected by hybridization under mild stringent conditions using HPV cocktail probes containing the 150 amplimer products of HPV 6, 11, 16, 18, 31, and 33. In addition HPV GP-PCR for identification of the individual

Table 3.2 Summary of commonly used general primers for HPV analyses

Authors	Primers	Region	Length of amplimer	Mechanism	HPV detected
Manos et al. 1989	My 09 My 11	L1	450 bp	Mixture HPV group/type specific primers	6, 11, 13, 16, 18–26, 30, 31, 33, 35, 39, 40, 42, 45, 51–57
Gregoire et al. 1989	IU IWDO	E1	850 bp	Mismatch acceptance (inosine)	6, 11, 16, 18, 33
Snijders et al. 1990	GP5 GP6	L1	150 bp	Mismatch acceptance	6, 11, 13, 16, 18, 30, 31, 33, 35, 39, 45, 51
van den Brule et al. 1990	GP1 GP2	E1	444 bp	Mismatch acceptance	same as Snijders

```
HPV  2a  TRSTN  VSLCA-TE----ASDTNYKATNFKE  Y L RH M EE
HPV  6b  TRSTN  MTLCAS-----VTTSSTYTNSDYKE  Y M RH V EE    32
HPV 11   TRSTN  MTLCAS-----VSKSATYTNSDYKE  Y M RH V EE
HPV 32   TRSTN  MTVCA-T----VTTEDTYKSTNFKE  Y L RH A EE
HPV 33   TRSTN  MTLC--TQ---VTSDSTYKNENFKE  Y I RH V EE
HPV 56   TRSTN  MTIS--T---ATEQLSKYDARKINQ  Y L RH V EE
HPV 57   TRSTN  VSLCA-T----VTTETNYKASNYKE  Y L RH M EE
HPV 58   TRSTN  MTLC--TE---VTKEGTYKNDNFKE  Y V RH V EE


HPV 16   TRSTN  MSLCAAI----STSETTYKNTNFKE  Y L RH G EE    33
HPV 31   TRSTN  MSVCAAI---A-NSDTTFKSSNFKE  Y L RH G EE
HPV 35   TRSTN  MSVCSA----VSSSDSTYKNDNFKE  Y L RH G EE
HPV 51   TRSTN  LTISTATA--AVS-P-TFTPSNFKQ  Y I RH G EE


HPV 13   TRSTN  MTVCAATT---SSLSDTYKATEYKQ  Y M RH V EE    34
HPV 18   TRSTN  LTICASTQ---SPVPGQYHATKFKQ  Y S RH V EE
HPV 39   TRSTN  FTLSTSIE---SSIPSTYDPSKFKE  Y T RH V EE
HPV 43   TRSTN  LTLCASTDPTV---PSTYDNAKFKE  Y L RH V EE
HPV 44   TRSTN  MTICAATTQ---SPPSTYTSEQYKQ  Y M RH V EE
HPV 45   TRSTN  LTLCASTQN---PVPSTYDPTKFKQ  Y S RH V EE
```

Fig. 3.5 Comparison of the putative amino acid sequence encoded by DNA fragments of the mucosotropic HPV types flanked by GP5/6 primer sequences.

HPV types positive samples will be subjected to a HPV type specific PCR (HPV-TS-PCR) for a limited number of HPV genotypes. GP-PCR positive samples which are negative by TS-PCR are considered to contain a previously unsequenced HPV genotype designated HPV-X.

GP 5/6 generates small fragments (150 bP). Therefore it is recommended to use this system for paraffin-embedded tissue since in this case smaller target DNA fragments can be expected due to fixation.

Since E6/E7 ORF are typically intact and transcriptionally active in neoplastic cells, some consensus systems have also been developed by the amplification of regions within the E6/E7 ORF. Unfortunately there is much divergence between genital HPV genotypes in this region making these systems less universal than the L1 and E1 region-based general primer method.

Recently an interesting observation has been made after sequencing of the GP5/6 PCR products of several genital HPVs. Translation of these sequences into the putative amino acid sequence according to the position of the L1 start codon and alignment of these amino acid sequences revealed the presence of strongly conserved amino acid residues at both ends of the GP-PCR products (see Fig. 3.5).

It appeared that all the mucosotropic HPVs contain the TRSTN amino acid sequence at the 5′ part of the GP-PCR product while the conserved pentamer RHXEE was found at the 3′ end (Van den Brule *et al.* 1992). These conserved sequences were not present in cellular sequences which were coamplified by these primers. In contrast, the internal region differing from 8 to 13 amino acid residues in length was found to be polymorphic.

Homology comparison of these unique HPV-GP-PCR sequences showed homology of more than 55 per cent at the nucleotide level with all known sequenced mucosotropic HPV types (kindly made available to us by Dr. H. Delius and Dr. L. Gissmann, DKFZ, Germany). Much lesser homology was observed with cellular and other viral sequences after databank searches.

Besides confirming viral specificity, the value of HPV GP-PCR product sequencing is the confirmation of homology between GP-PCR products derived from closely related HPV types; that is HPV 6 and 11 (84 per cent), HPV 18 and 45 (80 per cent), and HPV 33 and 58 (86 per cent). This is in agreement with a recently established phylogenetic study which revealed similar results using larger fragments of L1 and other ORF (Van den Brule *et al.* 1992).

Based on this knowledge the identification of novel HPVs seems to be possible by sequence analysis of HPV-GP-PCR generated products. This means that in addition to the application of HPV detection in epidemiological studies the HPV-GP-PCR can also be an important tool for the isolation of new HPV types.

3.2.5   Comparison of different HPV detection methods

In Table 3.3 the different HPV DNA detection methods are summarized.

A limited number of studies are reported on the comparison of Southern blot, ViraPap, and PCR results. In a case control study of cervical cancer in Spain and Columbia (Guerrero *et al.* 1992) the three different methods were applied and compared. The following results were obtained. Cervical scrapes of 510 women were tested, 237 samples (46.5 per cent) were negative in all tests performed. Using consensus PCR 40.4 per cent was positive. Applying SB and ViraPap only 17.8 per cent and 21.5 per cent showed HPV positivity respectively indicating the superiority of the PCR. The L1 consensus PCR detected many more HPV type 6, 11, 16, 18, 31, and 35 than ViraPap. ViraPap and SB sensitivity were similar. In a study designed by Schiffman *et al.* (1991), to compare L1 consensus primer PCR and SB 120 specimens were analysed. The two methods showed 80 per cent concordance and PCR was slightly more sensitive than Southern blotting. Discrepancy between these studies could be because in the case control study cervical smears were analysed while in the other study cervicovaginal lavage was used. This collecting method yields an increased DNA content which favours SB analysis but has the disadvantage of including both vaginal and cervical cells. This is in agreement with the general observation that HPV type specific PCR is more sensitive than SB, especially when the specimen size is limited. Another approach to evaluate the different HPV detection methods is to analyse its significance in epidemiological studies. Several case-control studies applying FISH, Southern blot, ViraPap or PCR have been reported. Variations between the HPV association and cervical cancer were obtained as reflected by differences in odds ratios (OR) and corresponding 95 per cent confidence intervals (CI). From these data it

Table 3.3 Short description and evaluation of HPV detection methods

Detection method	Material	Detection level (HPV copy/cell)	Advantages	Disadvantages
Filter *in situ* hybridization (FISH-spot blotting)	Lysed cells	10–100	Rapid Large numbers	Sensitivity 'insufficient'
Dot blotting	Isolated DNA	1–10	High specificity	Laborious
Southern blotting	Isolated DNA, Electro-phoresis	0.1–1 (using 5–10 μg if DNA)	Very high specificity	Very laborious
In situ hybridization[1]	Sections Cytospins	20	Preservation of morphology	Laborious
Polymerase chain reaction—DNA amplification method	Isolated DNA, Cell lysates, Sections	1 copy/sample	Rapid, Multiple detection, Extremely sensitive	Contamination, Separate rooms, Disposables

[1] Recently a PCR in situ hybridization has been developed and improvement of sensitivity can be expected (Nuovo *et al.* 1991. *Am. J. Pathol.* **139**, 1239.).

appeared that the weakest association (OR 2.1 CI 1.6–2.8) was found in the Costa Rica study and strongest association in the Columbia (OR 77.5 CI 10.6–568.0) and Spain (OR 45.3 CI 17.9–115.0) area. It appeared that the strongest associations were found with the more sensitive HPV detection methods like polymerase chain reaction, ViraPap, or Southern blot. The weaker associations were found with the less sensitive method filter *in situ* hybridization (FISH) (Munoz and Bosch 1992). Since large variations using the sensitive methods were found, it is clear that additional interassay comparisons are necessary. This will require a highly qualified reference centre(s) to establish standards for the different assays.

3.3 HPV prevalence rates in women with normal and abnormal cervices as detected by different HPV detection methods

3.3.1 Normal cervical epithelium

In Table 3.4 the results of some selected large HPV prevalence studies ($n > 90$) of normal cervical squamous epithelium are summarized. By using more HPV probes and PCR for HPV typing it appeared that a large variety of HPVs can be found. The most prevalent HPV type in these studies seems to be HPV 16. Since in most of these studies no colposcopy was done we do not know how many patients had actual lesions. HPV prevalence rates vary considerably. The highest HPV prevalence (33 per cent) was found in young women with multiple partners (Table 3.4, Bauer *et al.* 1991) showing that epidemiological risk factors for cervical cancer are strongly associated with genital HPV infections. In general a HPV prevalence between 10 and 20 per cent is found in young women visiting general hospitals or family planning clinics. In addition, in cervical cancer screening populations, a HPV positivity of 11.5–18.1 per cent is found in young women (see Table 3.4, Toon *et al.* 1986; Rohan *et al.* 1991) while in women over the age of 35 a lower HPV prevalence (1.5–3.5 per cent) was observed (see Table 3.4, Melcher *et al.* 1988; Van den Brule *et al.* 1991). This suggests an age dependency of HPV infections.

Recently we have studied the HPV prevalence rate in women between 15 and 55 years old in cytomorphologically normal smears. Comparing a group of women visiting a general hospital and a group of women visiting general practitioners it appeared in five-year-interval analysis that no differences existed. HPV 16 prevalence reached a maximum between 20 and 25 years but did not exceed 10 per cent. In both populations a gradual decrease in HPV positivity from 25 per cent to less than 5 per cent was observed. HPV 16 levels of about 1 per cent were reached after the age of 35 years. The results of the HPV age dependency of the hospital group

Table 3.4 HPV prevalence in cytologically normal cervical scrapes

Reference	n	Method	Population	Age in years	% HPV	HPV type	Area
1	1271	DB	screening	35–55	1.6	6,11,16,18	the Netherlands
2	215	DB	FPC/STD	± 28	19.5	16,18	UK
3	661	ViraPap	FPC/STD	13–19	15	6,11,16,18,31,33,35	USA
4	96	SB	general hospital	± 27.6	12.5	6,11,16,18,X	Germany
5	289	SB	general hospital	34	10	group 6[d] , group 31[e] , 16,18	USA
6	104	SB	screening	29.1	11.5	6,11,16,18	UK
7	1346	PCR[b]	screening	35–55	3.5	6,11,16,18,31,33,X	the Netherlands
8	593	PCR[b]	hospital	16–60	14	6,11,16,18,31,33,X	the Netherlands
9	467	PCR[a]	students	22.9	33[f]	6,11,16,18,31,33,35,39,45,52,X	USA
10	105	PCR[c]	screening	23	18.1	6,11,16,18,X	Canada

DB = DNA blot; SB = Southern blot; PCR[a] Myo9/11, Manos et al.; PCR[b] GP 5/6, Snijders et al.; PCR[c] IU/IWD0, Gregoire et al.; d = HPV 6, 11, 42, 42; e = HPV 31,33,35,39,45,51,52 and 56; X = unidentified HPV; f = calculated for cervical smears; FPC = family planning clinic; STD = sexual transmitted disease clinic.

References: 1. Melchers et al. 1988. J. Med. Virol., **25**, 11–16; 2. Wickenden et al. 1987. J. Pathol., **153**, 127–35; 3. Mosicki et al. 1987. Ped. Res., **28**, 507–513; 4. Schneider et al. 1987. Int. J. Cancer, **40**, 198–204; 5. Lorincz et al. 1990. Am. J. Obstet. Gynecol., **162**, 645–51; 6. Toon et al. 1986. Br. Med. J., **293**, 1261–64; 7. Van den Brule et al. 1991. Int. J. Cancer, **48**, 404–8; 8. ibid; 9. Bauer et al. 1991. JAMA, **265**, 472–77; 10. Rohan et al. 1991. Int. J. Cancer, **49**, 856–60.

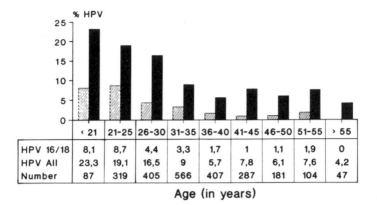

Fig. 3.6 Relationship between HPV prevalence in cytomorphologically normal cervical smears and age as detected in a general hospital population. GP 5/6 general HPV PCR in combination with HPV 16/18 TS PCR was applied. HPV include all PV GP-PCR positivity smears. Data are modified from Melkert *et al. Int. J. Cancer* 1993, **53**, 919–23.

is shown is Fig. 3.6. From these data it seems that HPV infections can be cleared in young and asymptomatic women and are often transient. Although less probable, a cohort effect cannot be excluded. The existence of transient HPV infections are also suggested by the observation that the presence of HPV 16 DNA can fluctuate in cytologically normal scrapes analysing consecutive smears after frequently sampling (Schneider *et al.* 1992). Interestingly HPV fluctuation (presence, absence, presence, etc.) and clearance has been found in young women with cytologically normal smears indicating that this phenomenon is clinically not important. HPV fluctuation in cervical smears with normal cytology from older women is yet to be investigated. The influence of fluctuation on HPV 16 prevalence rates can be minimized by studying large cohorts ($n > 1000$). Using this approach the 'running mean' of the prevalence rate of women with a HPV positive smear will be obtained. Since a HPV 16 prevalence of about 1 per cent in a large cohort of women older than 35 years ($n = 1346$, Table 3.4, Van den Brule *et al.* 1991) was found HPV fluctuation had taken place in only a minority of these cases. This dynamic character of HPV infection has consequences for the calculation of the proportion of HPV 16 infected women which eventually develop cervical cancer. Follow-up studies of women with normal cytology with either HPV negative or HPV positive smears has to be carried out to get insight in this problem.

From the HPV prevalence data in normal cytology reported to date it can be concluded that the large differences are most probably due to: (a) the HPV detection method used (see Section 3.2), and (b) poor definition of the cohort studied. It seems that age and sexual activity are the most important determinants of a cohort definition.

3.3.2   Premalignant and malignant cervical lesions

To understand and compare the results of different studies the relationship between different cytological and histological terms has to be explained (see also Chapter 1).

Cervical lesions which may progress to invasive carcinoma were initially histologically designated as dysplasia. Dysplasia is characterized by abnormal differentiation of cervical epithelium. Gradually lack of differentiation and increasing cellular atypia were suggested to be a hallmark for the development of cervical cancer. Dysplasia is divided into mild, moderate, and severe, depending on the proportion of the thickness of squamous epithelium with abnormal differentiation as shown by the disturbances of tissue architecture and the presence of atypical cells. Full thickness involvement is called carcinoma *in situ*. Richart (1968) proposed that the dysplastic changes represent a spectrum of the same basic change in cervical intra-epithelial neoplasia (CIN-concept). It was suggested that squamous cell carcinomas of the cervix develop through a continuum of progressive consecutive CIN lesions. Grade 1 (CIN I) represents atypical cells of the basal part of the epithelial layer up to one third of the total thickness, grade 2 one to two thirds, and grade 3 two thirds to whole thickness. Grade 3 also includes carcinoma *in situ*.

The Pap classification is used to characterize cytomorphological abnormalities in cervical smears. Pap I and II correspond to no significant morphological changes; Pap IIIa to mild to moderate dysplasia; Pap IIIb to severe dysplasia; Pap IV to carcinoma *in situ*; and Pap V to invasive carcinoma. The main drawback in histological classification and Pap smear reporting is the great inter- and intra-observer variation as scored by the pathologist. In an attempt to solve the problem of poor inter- and intra-pathologist reproducibility in 1988 the Bethesda classification system was introduced. Cervical intra-epithelial neoplasia (CIN) was replaced by squamous intra-epithelial lesion (SIL). It was proposed to classify CIN II and III as high-grade squamous intra-epithelial lesions (HSIL) and CIN I by low-grade squamous intra-epithelial lesions (LSIL). In the proposed SIL classification it was suggested that low-grade SIL lesions are not necessarily precursors of cervical cancer which either regress or persists but do not progress while high-grade SIL lesions were considered as one entity who progressed to cervical cancer. The relationship between Pap classification, dysplasia, CIN, and SIL is demonstrated in Fig. 3.7.

Several combined cyto-histological and HPV detection studies, using biopsies and cervical smears, have been carried out to investigate HPV prevalence of women with premalignant lesions. Here we have chosen to

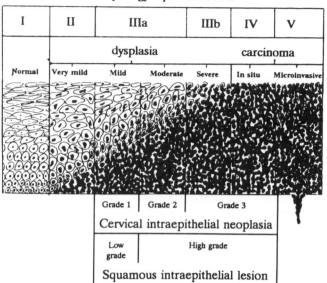

Fig. 3.7 Relationship between cervical dysplasia, cervical intra-epithelial neoplasia, and squamous intra-epithelial lesion. The cytological equivalents according to the Pap classification are also depicted.

present only the data of four large representative studies in which updated HPV detection methods, that is, Southern blot analysis and/or PCR, were used and which were recently performed.

In France, Bergeron *et al.* (1992) analysed low (CIN I) and high CIN lesions (CIN II + III) using mainly SB technique and 13 different HPV probes. In a substantial number of specimens PCR was also applied. Moreover, in many lesions HPV presence could also be confirmed by *in situ* hybridization.

Lungu *et al.* (1992) studied a total of 276 samples including CIN I, II, and III lesions using PCR with L1 consensus primers for HPV detection and RFLP analysis of PCR products for HPV typing.

In the Netherlands a large study was carried out (Van den Brule *et al.* 1991) using GP 5/6 primer mediated PCR in combination with HPV type specific PCR. Using cervical scrapes ($n = 835$) HPV prevalence rates were determined in cytomorphological abnormal smears categorized as Pap IIIa, Pap IIIb, and Pap IV equivalent to CIN I, II, and III respectively.

Lorincz *et al.* (1992) have screened for the presence of HPV DNA in cervical biopsies of CIN lesions and smears by low-stringency Southern blot (590 cervical samples). Positive samples were tested at high stringency

Table 3.5 An overview of four HPV prevalence studies in women with premalignant cervical disease as selected by biopsies and abnormal (> PapIII) cervical smears

Ref	Method		Classification	n	% HPV pos	6/11	16	18	30	31	33	35
1	SB +	B	Low CIN (1)	48	41 (85.4%)	–	20.8	2.1	4.2	–	4.2	2.1
	[a]PCR		High CIN (2+3)	53	49 (92.4%)	–	56.6	3.8	–	1.9	1.9	3.8
2	[b]PCR	B	CIN 1	100	91 (91%)	15	16	3		16	–	2
			CIN 2	74	74 (100%)	0.4	64.8	5.4		4.1	9.5	–
			CIN 3	102	102 (100%)	–	73.1	2		3	6	1
3	[c]PCR	S	PAPIIIa ~ CIN 1	588	435 (74%)	1.7	29.0	5.4		6.0	3.4	0.3
			PAPIIIb ~ CIN 2	177	141 (80%)	1.7	42.9	9.0		2.8	2.3	0.6
			PAPIV ~ CIN 3	70	70 (100%)	1.4	51.4	10		7.6	5.7	–
4	SB	B +	LSIL ~ CIN 1	377	262 (69%)	16.7	16.2	4.0		5.0	3.4	2.7
		S	HSIL ~ CIN 2 & 3	261	228 (87.3%)	3.1	47.1	5.0		10.3	4.6	4.2

SB = Southern blot; B = biopsies; S = smears; [a]Consensus PCR, Kawashima *et al*. 1990 *J. Invest. Dermatol*., **95**, 537–2; [b]Consensus PCR My09/My11 + RFLP, Manos *et al*. 1989; [c]GP/TS-PCR, van den Brule *et al*. 1990 *J. Clin. Microbiol*., **28**, 2739–43; X = unidentified; M = multiple infection; nm = not mentioned.

References: 1. Begeron *et al*. 1992. *Am. J. Surg. Pathol*., **16**, 641–49; 2. Lungu *et al*. 1992. *JAMA*, **267**, 2493–96; 3. Van den Brule *et al*. 1991. *Int. J. Cancer*, **48**, 404–8 + additional data; 4. Lorincz *et al*. 1992. *Obstet. Gynecol*., **79**, 328–37.

with specific probes for HPV 6/11, 16, 18, 31, 33, 35, 42, 43, 44, 45, 51, 52, 56, and 58.

From all these data summarized in Table 3.5 it is clear that, from a virologic point of view, CIN represents a heterogeneous disease. The main general observations are that the prevalence of HPV 16, 18 increases about twofold between CIN I and CIN II/III, whereas in the same lesions the prevalence of HPV 6/11, unidentified HPV types, and the presence of more than one HPV type (multiple infections) decreases. In Table 3.6 HPV prevalence rates in cervical squamous cell carcinoma of six large studies are summarized. It appeared that HPV prevalence rates vary between 84 and 100 per cent. In all these studies Southern blot and/or PCR was used. HPV 16/18 was the most prevalent virus (67–72 per cent) found in all the studies. There is a considerable variation between HPV 16 and 18 in the different study groups, for example the proportion of HPV 16 to HPV 18 in the US study was 2 to 1, while in a study in the Netherlands and India this proportion seems to be 10 to 1. This could indicate large variations in HPV 16 and 18 prevalences in different areas and needs further

	% HPV types														
39	40	42	43	44	45	51	52	56	57	58	59	61	66	X	M
10.4		–			2.1	12.5	2.1	6.3		4.2	–	2.1	–	25	
–		–			–	–	3.8	1.9		–	–	1.9	–	20.8	
					1	2			4					19	22
					–	1.4			–					4.1	9.5
					–	1			–					4	6
	0.2					0.9		1.0		2.6				16.8	6.6
	–					0.6		0.6		–				13.0	5.0
	–					1.4		2.8		1.4				11.3	7.1
			1.1	1.1	1.3	1.1	2.4	1.9	2.1	1.3				9.3	nm
			0.4	0	0.8	0.4	1.9	2.3	1.1	0.4				5.7	nm

clarification. Also the percentage of HPV negative carcinomas is not clear because different groups apply different detection techniques but the association between specific HPV types and cervical cancer is very high (Table 3.6). Exchange of HPV negative carcinoma samples between the different groups is necessary to solve the problem whether HPV negative cervical carcinomas exist.

Based on the HPV prevalence rates found in different CIN grades and cervical cancer, it was suggested by Lorincz *et al.* (1992) to divide HPV types in four different categories; that is, the low-risk HPV 6 group (HPV 6, 11, 42, 43, and 44), the intermediate-risk HPV 31 group (HPV 31, 33, 35, 52 and 58), the high-risk HPV 16 group, and the high-risk HPV 18 group (18, 45, 56). Taking all the data of summarized large studies in Tables 3.5 and 3.6 together it appears also that:

(1) the low-risk HPV 6 group is most frequently present in low grade CIN and (almost) absent in cancer;

(2) the intermediate-risk HPV 31 group is rather frequently detected in the high-grade CIN but in a rather low percentage of cervical cancer;

(3) the high-risk HPV 16 group is almost equally associated with CIN II and III and cervical cancer;

(4) the high-risk HPV 18 group is found in a relatively high number of invasive but less in CIN II and III lesions. This suggests that the HPV 18 group should be considered the most aggressive oncogenic type.

Table 3.6 HPV prevalence in cervical cancer

Ref	Method	n	% HPV pos	6/11	16	18	31	33	35	45	51	52	56	58	X	M	Area
1	SB	153	137 (89%)	–	47.1	23.5	1.3	1.3	1.3	2.0	0.7	0.7	1.3	1.3	5.2	nm	USA
2	PCR	120	120 (100%)	–	73.3	7.5	1.7	0.8							5.8	17	the Netherlands
3	PCR[b] + SB	96	94 (97.9%)	1.0	63.5	3.1	–	–	–						30.2	nm	India
4	PCR[a] + SB	53	47 (88.6%)	–	37.7	32.1	–	–		5.7					13.2	nm	East Africa
5	PCR[c]	29	29 (100%)	–	75.9	17.2	3.4	3.4		–					–	nm	USA
6	SB + PCR[d]	106	89 (83.9%)	–	54.7	12.3		6.6							10.4	nm	France

X = unclassified HPV types; M = multiple infections; SB = Southern blot; [a] = GP/TS PCR; [b] = TS–PCR; [c] = My09/11 PCR; [d] = TS–PCR; nm = not mentioned.

References: 1. Lorincz *et al.* 1992. *Obstet. Gynecol.*, **79**, 328–37; 2. Van den Brule, 1991. *Int. J. Cancer*, **48**, 404–8 + additional data; 3. Das *et al.* 1992. *J. Med. Virol.*, **36**, 329–45; 4. Ter Meulen *et al.* 1992. *Int. J. Cancer*, **51**, 515–21; 5. Resnick *et al.* 1990. *J. Natl. Cancer Inst.*, **82**, 1477–84; 6. Riou *et al.* 1990. *Lancet*, **335**, 1171–4.

Using the knowledge of possible HPV involvement in the development of cervical cancer the new classification system for pre-malignant lesions, that is, squamous intra-epithelial lesion (SIL) can be criticized (the 1988 Bethesda system for reporting cervical/vaginal cytologic diagnosis: developed and approved at the National Cancer Institute Workshop in Bethesda, Maryland, December 12–13, 1988. *Human Pathology* **21**, 704–8). It was proposed to replace CIN I by low-grade SIL (LSIL) with presumed little or no progression potential, while CIN II and III were considered as one entity called high SIL with a high progression potential. This hypothesis, however, is controversial. The presence of high-risk as well as intermediate- and low-risk HPV types in LSIL lesions and the association of high-risk types with cervical cancer suggests LSIL lesions can also progress to invasive cervical carcinomas. This implies that LSIL lesions are heterogeneous in their clinical behaviour, which is in contrast to the assumptions of the Bethesda classification. This is also confirmed by data from follow-up studies of women with HPV 16 positive smears and low-grade CIN lesions which show progression in a substantial number of cases to CIN III (Campion *et al.* 1986). This is in agreement with the observation that the type of HPV infection may influence the clinical outcome of a cervical lesion, that is, regression, persistance, or progression (Kataja *et al.* 1992).

Recently a new classification system of HPVs using phylogenetic or evolutionary trees based on amino acid and nucleotide sequence alignment data of the E6 ORF has been published (Van Ranst *et al.* 1992). The genital HPV types could be divided in three distantly related groups. It appeared that HPV 6, 11 13, 42, 43, 44, HPV 16, 31, 33, 35, 51, 52, 56, 58, and HPV 18, 45, and 39 belonged to three distinct phylogenetic trees. Since HPV grouping based on sequence homology and its biological behaviour (Lorincz *et al.* 1992) seems to be in good agreement, this knowledge needs to be incorporated in HPV testing using PCR. For example, optimal primer sets for the different risk groups could be composed. Although further research on the correlation between the presence of the different HPV types and disease progression is necessary, classification in HPV groups with different biological behaviour instead of individual HPV typing is less confusing and will be appreciated by the clinician.

3.4 Possible clinical implications

From the above-mentioned data it is unclear for the clinician which prognostic parameter he or she can use for the treatment of cervical lesions. Neither the CIN classification, nor the Pap smear, nor colposcopy can be used to assess the prognosis of an individual patient. So two main questions still remain. Can HPV typing of pre-malignant cervical lesions be used as

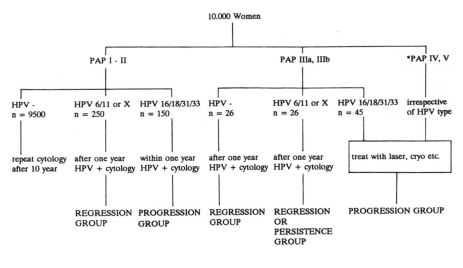

* All HPV positive

Fig. 3.8 HPV positivity in relation to cytological analysis of 10 000 cervical smears from a general population based cervical cancer programme of women older than 35 years.

a progression marker for individual management of the patient and is it possible to introduce HPV typing as a screening marker for cervical cancer screening?

Concerning cervical cancer screening it is necessary to compare HPV prevalence rates with cytomorphological results of cervical cancer screening programmes in countries which have developed a good cancer registration system. Population-based cervical cancer screening programs for women between 35 and 55 years using Pap smears have been carried out for nearly two decades in the Netherlands. From these programmes a large number of cytological data have been collected from the general population. Based on our 16 years of experience it appeared that 99 per cent of the women will have normal Pap smears (Pap I/II). From the 1 per cent with abnormal cytology 0.7 per cent will have Pap IIIa (mild dysplasia) and 0.27 per cent will have severe dysplasia (Pap IIIb). Carcinoma *in situ* (Pap IV) and cervical cancer (Pap V) will be found in 0.03 per cent of this population. During the last years routine cytological smears have been analysed and simultaneously HPV detection has been performed by PCR in this well-defined population. Smears ($n = 2227$) were collected from three cohorts of asymptomatic women participating in a triennial screening programme (1987, 1988, 1989) in an area with a low cervical cancer incidence. Abnormal smears were collected from the same cohorts and supplemented with abnormal smears from a university and a general hospital. The results of HPV prevalence rates using the HPV GP/TS-PCR strategy are summarized in Tables 3.5 and 3.6. In the cytologically normal smears of the asymptomatic women an overall HPV prevalence of 4 per cent was found. The frequencies of HPV type 16, 18, 31, and 33 was 1.5 per cent. In smears with mild ($n = 583$) and severe ($n = 177$) dysplasia and smears with carcinoma *in situ* ($n = 78$) the overall HPV prevalence was 74, 80, and 100 per cent respectively.

HPV 16, 18, 31, and 33 rates increased from 43 to 57 and 80 per cent in mild and severe dysplasia and carcinoma *in situ* respectively. In all cervical carcinomas ($n = 120$) HPV DNA was detected.

By comparing Pap smear results and the expected HPV prevalence, the value of HPV detection in cervical cancer screening can now be be evaluated (Meijer *et al.* 1992). Based on a population of 10 000 women the distributions of the different HPV genotypes over the different Pap classes are given in Fig. 3.8. The following screening scenarios would be possible.

1. HPV testing could be used as a *preselection* for women to undergo cytological examination (Pap smears). The shortcomings of HPV testing as a preselection for Pap test are HPV negative Pap IIIa ($n = 21$) and Pap IIIb ($n = 5$) will not be detected in a population of 10 000 women. Although there are indications from ongoing follow-up studies (Meijer *et al.* 1992) that no progression can be found in the absence of HPV, progression of HPV negative Pap III a and b cannot be completely excluded at this moment. Moreover, although we think that HPV negative cervical carcinomas are rare, there is still not enough evidence that all cervical carcinomas are HPV positive and this may be missed in screening programmes. This will give resistance by cytologists and clinicians to use a prescreening step for cervical cancer. However, it has to be considered that Pap smears are missing at least 10 per cent of the cervical carcinomas (Koss 1989).

Therefore we favour another scenario.

2. This is HPV testing in combination with cytology. The advantage of this approach is that abnormal cytology and cervical cancer will not be missed. However, in population screening programs the overwhelming majority of scrapes (9500 out of 10 000) will be cytomorphologically and HPV negative. Moreover, from epidemiological studies it is clear that the time to develop an invasive cervical carcinoma for a woman with a normal cervical smear lasts at least 12 to 13 years (report population screening cervical cancer, 1989, Institute for Social Health Care, Erasmus University, Rotterdam, the Netherlands). This offers an advantage in terms of screening since in the double (cytology and HPV detection) negative cases, the Pap smear interval could be extended from

three years (presently performed in the Netherlands) to eight or even ten years. In this scenario it would even be possible to consider a reduction in the population-based cervical cancer screening of women over 35 years to every decade.

Figure 3.8 also includes a possible advice for patient management. For women with cytomorphologically normal smears but containing oncogenic HPV types, the cytology and HPV testing should be repeated within one year. This is because because they may belong to the progression group since they possibly have a persistent HPV infection. Women with HPV 6/11 and X should also be followed up for one year to ensure that they remain cytological negative. It is suggested that women which are positive for oncogenic HPV types and show abnormal cytology ≥ Pap IIIa belong to the progression group and have to be treated (laser, cryo, loop, etc.). The group Pap IIIa and b with HPV negative smears or non-oncogenic HPV types should be followed up after one year by HPV testing and cytology and but need not be treated. When screening HPV negative and cytological negative they can be included in the newly proposed population-based screening strategy. This approach of different treatment strategies for women with HPV negative or non-oncogenic HPV types could be very useful for the clinician because it relates directly the presence of oncogenic HPV types to prognosis and prevents overtreatment of these lesions. Although there are already indications that women with cytomorphologically abnormal and HPV negative smears do not show progression of their cervical lesion, well-defined follow-up studies of women with HPV positive or negative smears with abnormal cytology has been carried out to confirm our hypothesis based on extensive preliminary observations in on-going follow-up studies of CIN lesions. The benefits of HPV screening in combination with cytology would be:

(1) strong reduction of screening of women over the age of 35 years —screening every eight or ten years resulting in a substantial reduction of screening cost which is at present made by triennial screening using the Pap smear alone;

(2) saving costs for colposcopy and gynaecological treatment of patients with Pap IIIa or IIIb who do not have oncogenic HPV types.

Acknowledgements

The authors thank Miss Yvonne Duiker and Miss Carla van Rijn for excellent preparation of the manuscript and dr. P. van der Valk for critical reading. This work was in part supported by the Dutch Cancer Society, Koningin Wilhelmina Fonds: Grants IKA-VU 91–17; IKA-VU-93–605 and the Prevention Fund, the Netherlands Grant 28–1502.

References

Bauer, H. M., Ting, Y. Greer, C. E. *et al.* (1991). Genital human papillomavirus infection in female university students as determined by a PCR-based method. *JAMA*, **265**, 472–77.

Bergeron, C., Barrasso, R., Beaudenon, S., Flamant, P., Croissant, O., and Orth, G. (1992). Human papillomaviruses associated with cervical intra-epithelial neoplasia. *American Journal of Surgical Pathology*, **16**, 641–9.

Brandsma, J., Burk, R. D., Lancaster, W. D., Pfister, H., and Schiffman, M. H. (1989). Interlaboratory variation as an explanation for varying prevalence estimates of human papillomavirus infection. *International Journal of Cancer*, **43**, 260–2.

Brigati, D. J., Meyerson, D., Leavy, J. J. Spalholz, B., Travis, S. Z., Fong, C. K. *et al.* (1983). Detection of viral genomes in cultured cells and paraffin embedded tissue sections using biotin labelled hybridization probes. *Virology*, **126**, 32–50.

Campion, M. J., McCance, D. J., Cuzick, J., and Singer, A. (1986). Progressive potential of mild cervical atypia: prospective cytological and virological study. *Lancet*, **2**, 237–40.

De Villiers, E. M. (1989). Heterogeneity of human papillomavirus group. *Journal of Virology*, **63**, 4808–903.

Ehrlich, H. A., Gelfland, H. A., and Sninsky, J. J. (1991). Recent advances in the polymerase chain reaction. *Science*, **252**, 1643–51.

Gissmann, L. and Schneider, A. (1986). The role of human papillomaviruses in genital cancer. In: *Herpes and papillomaviruses. Their role in the carcinogenesis of the lower genital tract.* (eds. G. de Palo, F. Rilkes, and H. zur Haussen). Raven Press, New York, Vol. 31, pp.15–25.

Gregoire, L., Arella, M., Campione-Piccardo, J., and Lancaster, W. D. (1989). Amplification of human papillomavirus DNA sequences by using conserved primers. *Journal of Clinical Microbiology*, **27**, 2660–5.

Guerrero, E., Daniel, R. W., Bosch, F. X. Castellsague, X., Munoz, N., Gili, M. *et al.* (1992). Comparison of ViraPap, southern hybridization and polymerase chain reaction methods for human papillomavirus identification in an epidemiological investigation of cervical cancer. *Journal of Clinical Microbiology*, **30**, 2951–9.

Kataja, V., Syrjänen, S., Mantyjävir, R., Yliskoski, M., Saarikoski, S., and Syrjänen, K. (1992). Prognostic factors in cervical human papillomavirus infections. *Sexually Transmitted Diseases*, **19**, 154–60.

Koss, L. S. (1989). The Papanicolaou test for cervical cancer detection: a triumph and a tragedy. *Journal of the American Medical Association*, **261**, 737–43.

Longo, M. C., Berninger, M. S., and Hartley, J. L. (1990). Use of uracil DNA glycolase to control carry-over contamination in polymerase chain reactions. *Genes*, **93**, 125–8.

Lorincz, A. T., Reid, R., Jenson, A. B., Greenberg, M. D., Lancaster, W. D., and Kurman, R. J. (1992). Human papilloamvirus infection of the cervix: Relative risk associations of fifteen common anogenital types. *Obstetrics Gynecology*, **79**, 328–37.

Manos, M. M., Wright, D. K., Lewis, A. J. D., Broker, T. R., and Wolinsky, S. M. (1989). The use of polymerase chain reaction amplification for the detection of genital human papillomavirusis. In *Molecular diagnostics of human cancer* (eds. M. Furth and M. Greaves), pp. 209–14, Molecular Diagnostics of Human Cancer. Cancer Cells 7, Cold Spring Harbor Press, Cold Spring Harbor, NY.

Meijer, C. J. L. M., Van den Brule, A. J. C., Snijders, P. J. F., Helmerhorst, Th., Kenemans, P., and Walboomers, J. M. M. (1992). Detection of human papillomavirus in cervical scrapes by the polymerase chain reaction in relation to cytology: possible implications for cervical cancer screening. In *The epidemiology of cervical cancer and human papillomavirus*, pp. 271–281. IARC, Lyon, France.

Meisels, A. and Morin, B. (1981). Human papillomavirus and cancer of the uterine cervix. *Gynecologic Oncology*, **12**, 111–23.

Melchers, W. G. J., Herbrink, P. Quint, W. G. V. Walboomers, J. M. M., Meijer, C. J. L. M. and Lindeman , J. (1988). Prevalence of genital HPV infections in a regularly screened population in the Netherlands in relation to cervical cytology. *Journal of Medical Virology*, **25**, 11–16.

Mullis, K. B. and Faloona, F. A. (1987). Specific synthesis of DNA *in vitro* via a polymerase analyzed chain reaction. *Methods in Enzymology*, **155**, 335–50.

Munoz, N. and Bosch, F. X. (1992). HPV and cervical cancer: Review of case control and cohort studies. In *The epidemiology of human papilloma virus and cervical cancer* (eds. N. Munoz, F. X. Bosch, K. V. Shah, and A. Meheus), pp. 251–63. IARC publication no. 119, Lyon, France.

Richart, R. M. (1968). Natural history of cervical intra-epithelial neoplasia. *Clinical Obstetrics Gynecology*, **10**, 748–84.

Rohan, T., Mann, V., McLaughlin, J., Harnish, D. G., Yu, H., Smith, D., Davis, R., Shier, R. M., and Rawls, W. (1991). PCR-detected genital papillomavirus infection: prevalence and association with risk factors for cervical cancer. *International Journal of Cancer*, **49**, 856–60.

Rotkin, L. D. (1967). Adolescent coitus and cervical cancer: association of related events with increased risk. *Cancer Research*, **27**, 603–17.

Schiffman, M. H., Bauer, M., Lorincz, A. T. Manos, M. M., Byrne, J. C., Glass, A. G. *et al*. (1991). Comparison of southern blot hybridization and polymerase chain reaction methods for the detection of human papillomavirus DNA. *Journal of Clinical Microbiology*, **29**, 573–7.

Schneider, A., Krichhoff, T., Meinhardt, G., and Gissmann, L. (1992). Repeated evaluation of human papillomavirus 16 status in cervical swabs of young women with a history of normal papnicolaou smears. *Obstetrics Gynecology*, **79**, 683–88.

Snijders, P. J. F., Van den Brule, A. J. C., Schrijnemakers, H. F. J., Snow, G., Meijer, C. J. L. M., and Walboomers, J. M. M. (1990). The use of general primers in the polymerase chain reaction permits the detection of a broad spectrum of human papillomavirus genotypes. *Journal of General Virology*, **71**, 173–81.

Stoler, M. H., Rhodes, C. R., Whitbeck, A., Chow, L. T., and Broski, T. R. (1990) Gene expression of HPV types 16 and 18 in cervical neoplasia. In *Papillomaviruses* (eds. P. M. Howley, T. R. Broker), pp. 1–11. Wiley Liss, New York.

Syränen, K. and Syränen, S. (1989). Concept of the existence of human papillomavirus (HPV) DNA in histologically normal squamous epithelium of the genital tract should be re-evaluated. *Acta Obstetrics Gynecology Scandinavia*, **68**, 613–17.

The 1988 Bethesda system for reporting cervical/vaginal cytologic diagnosis: Developed and approved at the National Cancer Institute Workshop in Bethesda, Maryland, December 12–13, 1988. *Human Pathology*, **21**, 704–8.

Toon, P. G. Arrand J. R., Wilson, L. P., and Sharp, D. S. (1986). Human papillomavirus infection of the uterine cervix of women without cytological signs of neoplasia. *British Medical Journal*, **293**, 1261–4.

Van den Brule, A. J. C., Claas, H. C. J., Du Maine, M. Melchers, W. J. G., Helmerhorst, T. Quint, W. G. V. *et al.* (1989). Use of anticontamination primers in the polymerase chain reaction for the detection of human papillomavirus genotypes in cervical scrapes and biopsies. *Journal of Medical Virology*, **29**, 20–7.

Van den Brule, A. J. C., Meijer, C. J. L. M., Bakels, V., Kenemans, P., and Walboomers, J. M. M. (1990a). Rapid human papillomavirus detection in cervical scrapes by combined general primers mediated and type specific polymerase chain reaction. *Journal of Clinical Microbiology*, **28**, 2739–43.

Van den Brule, A. J. C., Snijders, P. J. F., Gordijn, R. L. J., Bleker, O. P., Meijer, C. J. L.M., and Walboomers, J. M. M. (1990b). General primer mediated polymerase chain reaction permits the detection of sequenced and still unsequenced human papillomavirus genotypes in cervical scrapes and carcinomas. *International Journal of Cancer*, **45**, 644–9.

Van den Brule, A. J. C., Walboomers, J. M. M., Maine, M. du, Kenemans, P., and Meijer C. J. L. M. (1991). Difference in prevalence of human papillomavirus genotypes in cyto morphologically normal cervical smears is associated with a history of cervical intra-epithelial neoplasia. *International Journal of Cancer*, **48**, 404–8.

Van den Brule, A. J. C., Snijders, P. J. F., Raaphorst, P., Schrijnemakers, H., Delius, H., Gissmann, L. *et al.* (1992). General primer PCR in combination with sequence analysis to identify potentially novel HPV genotypes in cervical lesions. *Journal of Clinical Microbiology*, **30**, 1716–21.

Van Ranst, M., Kaplan, J. B., and Burk, R. D. (1992). Phylogenetic classification of human papillomaviruses: correlation with clinical manifestations. *Journal of General Virology*, **73**, 2653–60.

Wagner, D., Ikenberg, H., Bohm, N., and Gissmann, L. (1984). Identification of human papillomavirus in cervical swabs by deoxyribomucleic acid *in situ* hybridization. *Obstetrics Gynecology*, **64**, 767–72.

Zur Hausen, H. (1977). Human papillomaviruses and their possible role in squamous cell carcinomas. *Current Topics Microbiology Immunology*, **78**, 1–30.

Zur Hausen, H. (1989). Papillomaviruses in anogenital cancer as a model to understand the role of viruses in human cancers. *Cancer Research*, **49**, 4677–81.

Zur Hausen, H. (1991). Human papillomaviruses in the pathogenesis of anogenital cancer. *Virology*, **184**, 9–13.

4 Epidemiology of HPV and cervical cancer

CIARAN WOODMAN

4.1 Introduction

Over the last 12 years a stream of imaginative and resourceful laboratory-based research has established an impressive, almost overwhelming, set of oncogenic credentials for human papilloma virus (HPV). So well has HPV prospered at the bench that there is now considerable enthusiasm for a vaccine development programme. This chapter does not attempt to reprise these exciting developments, which are dealt with elsewhere in the book, but rather to chronicle the efforts of epidemiologists and others to more precisely define the role of this virus in the etiology of squamous neoplasia and to illustrate where scientific uncertainty still persists. In an attempt to improve communication between epidemiologists, clinicians, and molecular biologists, more reference has been made than is usual to the basic principles which underpin the design and analysis of epidemiological enquiries of cervical neoplasia.

4.2 The evidence from case-control studies: General comments

In a case-control study, subjects are selected according to whether they do (cases) or do not (controls) have the disease under study. The groups are then compared with respect to the proportion having a history of exposure or characteristics of interest. The strength of the association between the exposure and the disease is measured by an odds ratio which may in certain circumstances provide a true measure of relative risk (Hennekens and Buring 1987). Valid estimates of the true association between exposure and disease depend on the selection of appropriate case and control groups. Cases should be defined according to explicit criteria and although there is usually little difficulty in distinguishing cases of invasive cervical cancer some investigators have taken the sensible precaution of using a pathology review panel to confirm the diagnosis (Muñoz *et al.* 1992). Case-control studies of cervical intra-epithelial neoplasia (CIN) are more problematic.

The difficulty arises from what are now frequently described as 'low grade' lesions. One such study includes among the case series women with cytological abnormality who were found on histological sampling to have 'koilocytotic atypia' alone (Morrison *et al.* 1991). As these histological changes are considered by many to be pathognomic of HPV infection, their inclusion will inevitably inflate measures of association (Morrison *et al.* 1991). It may also be difficult to distinguish the histological features of HPV infection from CIN1 and it would seem prudent to confine case-control studies of CIN to CIN2 and CIN3 lesions.

Cases may be drawn from a variety of sources. Hospital series provide the most convenient sampling frame. Population-based studies which include all or a random sample of cases occurring in a given time period in a defined population offer additional advantages (Muñoz *et al.* 1992; Reeves *et al.* 1989). They avoid the bias which may arise from whatever selection factors lead an affected individual to attend a specific institution. Hospital series may include an excess of screen-detected tumours or late stage disease dependent on whether it is primarily a surgical or radiotherapy facility. This may restrict the generalizability of studies conducted within these institutions. While incident or prevalent cases may be used, the former are always preferable. The defining characteristic of prevalent cases is their survival. Case-control comparisons using prevalent cases not only measure the antecedents of disease but also the determinants of survival. Inferences made on case-control studies using prevalent cases have, in the past, had to be revised when further studies were undertaken using incident cases (Rogentine *et al.* 1973). Although this is unlikely to be a major source of bias in studies of cervical neoplasia where the majority of tumours appear to be HPV positive, it is interesting to note that some investigators have reported that HPV positive tumours have a better prognosis although this is not a constant finding (DeBritton *et al.* 1993; Higgins *et al.* 1991; Riou *et al.* 1990).

The selection of an appropriate control group is equally important. Controls should be comparable to the source population from which the cases came. The use of general population controls offers major advantages in this respect especially when a population-based series of cases has been used. Hospital controls are more accessible, more likely to participate and less likely to show recall bias. They, however, have one important disadvantage; their reasons for admission may include conditions which share common etiological factors with the disease under scrutiny. Case-control studies of CIN present an additional problem with choice of control group. It is customary to exclude from such comparisons subjects with any history of cytological abnormality. This on the face of it seems reasonable because it reduces the risk of misclassification of disease status. However, given the strong association of cytological abnormality with a history of HPV infection and the high prevalence of abnormal cervical smears in many populations, the exclusion of these subjects will possibly result in a substantial underestimate of the true prevalence of HPV in the control population and as a result spuriously inflate case-control differences.

4.3   Hospital-based case-control studies

The first of these was a small hospital-based case-control study undertaken in Birmingham, England. This described a weak association of cervical neoplasia with the finding of HPV 16 DNA sequences in histological material. A surprise finding in this study, in the light of results presented below, was that the prevalence of HPV 16 appeared to increase with age. When the analyses were adjusted for differences in the age structure of the cases and controls the association ceased to be significant (Meanwell *et al.* 1987). An even smaller case control study undertaken in Uganda reported a substantially greater risk associated with HPV infection (odds ratio = 22, 95 per cent confidence intervals (CI) 5.1, 104.3, Schmauz *et al.* 1989). The investigators also found, despite the small size of the study, a substantial and significant association of cervical neoplasia with antibodies to herpes simplex virus type 1 and/or antibodies to herpes simplex virus type 2. Smaller, but also significant associations, with antibodies to cytomegalovirus and the viral capsid antigen of Epstein Bar virus, were also revealed. A linear trend in the risk for cervical cancer was noted with increasing numbers of infection. The largest of the hospital base case control studies was undertaken in China. This reported an odds ratio of 32.9 (95 per cent CI 7.7, 141.1) when the polymerase chain reaction (PCR) was used to determine the prevalence of HPV 16 and HPV 33 DNA sequences in cases and controls (Peng *et al.* 1991). Although an odds ratio of 33 should not be lightly set aside, the validity of this estimate was undermined by the drawing of cases and controls from different areas. The majority of cases were drawn from an urban conurbation whereas the majority of controls came from the surrounding rural areas. This may in part explain why only 1 of 146 controls in the study were HPV 16 positive. In addition this study provides no information on the number of sexual partners and age of first coitus in cases and controls. The conservatism of Chinese society is offered as an explanation for failing to collect detailed information on sexual behaviour patterns.

4.4   Population-based case-control studies

There have been two large population base case-control studies. The first, from Brazil includes 759 cases and 1467 controls (Reeves *et al.* 1989). When filter *in situ* hybridization was used to compare the prevalence of

Table 4.1 Association between invasive cancer and HPV DNA (data from Mūoz *et al.* 1992)

Detection method	Spain OR (95 %CI)	Columbia OR (95 %CI)
ViraPap	29.1 (10.3,81.9)	93.2 (12.6,687.3)
Southern blot hybridization	8.8 (4.1,19)	9.6 (3.7,25.1)
PCR	46.2 (18.5,115.1)	15.6 (6.9,34.7)

OR = odds ratio

HPV DNA sequences in cases and controls a significant association of cervical neoplasia with HPV status was noted. The strength of this association increased with the intensity of the signal. An odds ratio of 9.1 (95 per cent CI 6.1, 13.6) was reported when only cases and controls showing a strong signal were compared. It has been suggested, not unreasonably, that this study might have demonstrated a much greater association if a more accurate viral detection system had been used.

However, the most important case-control study examining the HPV hypothesis has only recently been reported (Muñoz *et al.* 1992). This population-based case-control study, undertaken in Columbia and Spain, is of the highest quality. It fulfils many of the criteria for valid case-control comparisons which have been previously outlined. Cases and controls were selected and identified using explicit criteria; participation was high and a variety of detection systems used to determine viral status. It both deserves and demands critical scrutiny because relative risks of this magnitude in cancer epidemiology have not been described since the association between smoking and lung cancer was revealed.

Although the direction of the association is consistent across both countries, its magnitude varies (Table 4.1). This is not totally surprising given that Columbia has a very high incidence of cervical cancer and Spain an extremely low incidence. What is perhaps surprising is that the magnitude of the association varies with the detection system used and in a not entirely predictable manner. The odds ratio is substantially less in both societies when Southern blot (SB) hybridization is used but highest in Spain with use of the PCR and in Colombia with the ViraPap test.

This instability can in part be explained by the small number of positive controls, 19 in all, when the PCR is used. This may also explain

Table 4.2 Modification of risk estimates for cervical neoplasia with HPV infection by sample cellular DNA content (re-analysis of Guerrero et al. 1992)

Sample cellular content (ng)	Southern blot		ViraPap		PCR	
	Cases/controls	OR (95%CI)	Cases/controls	OR (95%)	Cases/controls	OR (95%)
<1000	56/3	22.6 (7.03,114.76)	72/12	9.4 (4.78,19.86)	68/9	28.2 (12.03,70.5)
1001–5000	99/18	8 (4.4,15)		5.7 (3.3,10)	59/7	25.0 (9.8,70)
>5000	69/13	2.8 (1.4,6.2)		2.9 (1.4,6.3)	58/5	15.6 (4.7,59)
Trend	$X_2MH = 10.56$ $p < 0.001$		$X_2MH = 10.68$ $p < 0.001$		$X_2MH = 5.86$ $p < 0.025$	

OR = odds ratio

why, although the incidence of invasive cancer is seven times higher in Colombia than in Spain, it is only with use of the PCR is a difference observed in the prevalence of HPV 16 between the respective control populations.

However, a subsequent publication which describes in detail the scientific methods used suggest a more serious concern (Guerrero *et al.* 1992). These data show that the proportion of HPV positive women increases with increasing amounts of cellular DNA in cytological samples taken from both cases and controls. This relationship between sample DNA content and HPV positivity is not a straightforward linear relationship and the rate of increase differs between cases and controls.

When the odds ratios describing the association between HPV status and cervical neoplasia are recalculated for each sample volume, the odds ratios are largest when the DNA volume is least and decrease as the volume increases (Table 4.2). A similar significant trend is seen for all three methods of viral detection. This is worrying because the overall estimate of risk will be affected by the relative proportion of small and large volume samples. If all samples were small, then large estimates of association would be observed; if all were large then, only small estimates would be reported. This is unsatisfactory. It is not a simple matter of random misclassification occurring when sample DNA volume is small or merely adjusting for different numbers of small volume DNA samples in cases and controls. Rather, it suggests differential misclassification at small volumes and as such cannot be controlled for in the analysis. One interpretation of these findings is that the presence of epithelial abnormality lowers the threshold for detection of HPV. Another interpretation would be that quantitative rather than qualitative differences in the level of HPV infection are being observed. Some support for this possibility is that the trend is least marked with the use of the PCR. This illustrates one of the major limitations of the case-control design, the temporal ambiguity surrounding the timing of exposure and onset of disease.

4.5   Cohort studies

These difficulties can only be overcome by cohort studies in which longitudinal observations are made on a group of subjects whose exposure status has been defined prior to the onset of disease. For example, a random sample of the population first stratified by HPV status and followed for such time until sufficient numbers had developed invasive cancer, would provide the answer. Such a study is ethically impossible and some investigators have used CIN3 as a surrogate endpoint and recruited cohorts of subjects who are likely to be at greater risk of reaching this endpoint.

4.6   Progression studies

Campion *et al.* described a prospective study of 100 women with recurrent mildly dyskariotic smears (Campion *et al.* 1986). 58 per cent of those positive for HPV 16 progressed to CIN3 within two years as compared to 20 per cent of those with HPV 6. Koutsky and colleagues recruited a cohort of 241 women with negative cytology who were attending a sexually transmitted disease clinic (Koutsky *et al.* 1992). Those who were HPV 16 or 18 positive were significantly more likely to progress to CIN2/3 (odds ratio = 11, 95 per cent CI 4.6, 26). Other independent predictors of progression in this study were a past history of gonorrhoeal infection and antibodies to CMV and chlamydia. We have used archival material and the PCR to examine the risk of progression in 96 patients who were allocated the non-intervention arm of a randomized controlled trial. All had histological evidence of HPV infection alone or in association with CIN1 or CIN2. Patients who were HPV 16 or 18 positive on their initial biopsy were significantly more likely to progress than those who were HPV negative. By 4 years 56 per cent of the HPV 16 positive cases had progressed compared to 25 per cent of the HPV negative group (95 per cent, CI on difference in proportion 10–48 per cent). Murthy and colleagues, using a nested case-control design within a large cohort study, again confirmed a significant risk of progression associated with the presence of HPV 16 or 18 DNA sequences (odds ratio = 5.9, 95 per cent CI 2.5, 14.1) (Murthy *et al.* 1990).

All progression studies share a number of methodological problems. Baseline disease status may be misclassified. This is more likely with a study which uses a cytological entry point but can still occur as a result of sampling error when a colposcopically directed punch biopsy provides a histological definition of baseline status. Also virological status may be wrongly assigned. However, if virological status, baseline disease, and follow-up status are independently defined, then these errors are likely to be random and as such will only underestimate the true risk of progression associated with HPV status. There is another more serious reservation. Although HPV may accelerate progression to CIN3, not all women with CIN3 will progress to invasive cancer. As we cannot yet distinguish those cases which will progress it might be unwise to infer from those data that HPV infection results in the inexorable progression of all CIN lesions to invasive cancer.

4.7   The determinants of genital HPV infection

4.7.1   Age and HPV infection

Irrespective of the population studied or the detection system used, cross-sectional and longitudinal inquiries suggest the prevalence of cervical HPV

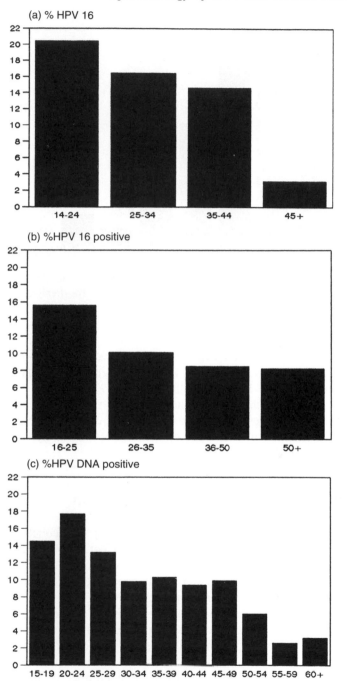

Fig. 4.1 Relationship between age and HPV infection in different countries: (a) Tanzania, (b) Basque Country, (c) Germany.

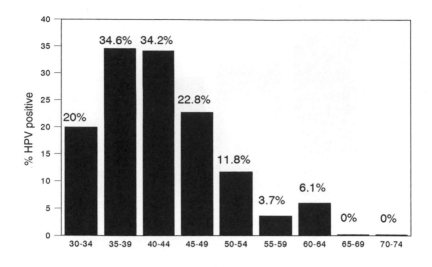

Fig. 4.2 HPV DNA positivity following hysterectomy for benign disease. (data from De Villiers *et al.* 1992)

infection declines with increasing age; a relationship that appears to hold across very different societies (Fig. 4.1) (Ter Meulen *et al.* 1992; Mugica-van Herckenrode *et al.* 1992; De Villiers *et al.* 1992).

So constant is this relationship that it survives the removal of the cervix. Figure 4.2 displays the age-specific prevalence of HPV DNA sequences in vaginal smears taken from women who have had a hysterectomy for benign disease (De Villiers *et al.* 1992).

4.8   Sexual behaviour and HPV infection

The first generation of case-control studies threw up a disconcerting finding. Sexual behaviour did not appear to predict cervical HPV infection (Reeves *et al.* 1989). A critical point, because the association of cervical neoplasia with certain sexual behaviour patterns has remained a constant finding of all substantial epidemiological inquiries.

HSV has an impeccable profile in this respect. Decreasing age at first coitus and increasing number of sexual partners are both associated with an increasing prevalence of antibody positive subjects (Hildesheim *et al.* 1991; Kjaer *et al.* 1990). Defining the link between sexual behaviour and HPV status has therefore been the focus of a number of inquiries. Some report positive findings. Ley and colleagues describe, in a young American college population, how the proportion of HPV positive cases increases significantly with number of lifetime sexual partners and decreasing age of first coitus (Ley *et al.* 1991). Rosenfield and colleagues describe a much weaker association and only then in teenagers (Rosenfeld *et al.* 1989). Moscicki *et al.* (1989) report that HPV positive women had a significantly greater number of sexual partners; women with more than 11 sexual partners had a three times greater risk of HPV infection than those who had less than three lifetime partners.

Others have reported negative, non-significant, or ambiguous results (Kiviat *et al.* 1989; Rohan *et al.* 1991; Van Doornum *et al.* 1992). Kjaer, in a population based case-control study of women from Denmark and Greenland, not only failed to demonstrate an association with age at first coitus but also reported that the risk of HPV 16/18 infection decreased significantly with increasing age (Kjaer *et al.* 1990). Burkett *et al.* (1992) found no association with number of sexual partners but a significant association with number of recent sexual episodes. Azocar reports that monogamous women are less likely to be HPV positive but the conclusion that sexual behaviour predicts infection is weakened by the absence of data stratifying HPV status by number of sexual partners and failure to demonstrate an association with age at first coitus (Azocar *et al.* 1990).

How can these incoherent findings be explained? The limitations of the test used for viral detection have been cited. Random misclassification following the use of an insensitive test will certainly attenuate any association. But even using a sensitive detection system, some have failed to show a relationship with sexual behaviour (Burkett *et al.* 1992). The age distribution of the populations studied varies. In a young population, acquisition of infection is studied; in an older population persistence of infection. In one, sexual behaviour may be important; in the other, this seems less likely. A serological test, such as antibody levels to HSV, provides a reliable and permanent measure of lifetime exposure. Cervical HPV infection is often a transient state and a one-sample test is almost certainly a poor reflection of ever having been exposed. It has also been suggested that persistent or repeated infection may suppress viral expression and reduce the likelihood of detection.

There is also the possibility that studies showing a positive association may be flawed. It is known that sexual behaviour predicts clinically overt disease, that is, genital warts. It is also known that sexual behaviour predicts subclinical infection, that is, cytological abnormalities. But the question remains, does it predict latent infection? Does it predict those women with no clinical disease, with negative cytology but detectable HPV DNA sequences? Burkett *et al.* (1992) present evidence to suggest that it does not. The investigators show that age at first coitus and number of sexual partners distinguish those with clinical and subclinical infection from those with no clinical or cytological abnormality. These variables, however, do not distinguish those with latent infection and those with no detectable DNA sequences.

The three studies which report a positive association with sexual behaviour may have confused the issue by including substantial numbers of women with clinical and sub-clinical disease. Only one acknowledges this possibility and asserts that the exclusion of these cases, which included 25 per cent of the sample and 38 per cent of the HPV positive cases made no difference to the observed relationship (data not shown) (Ley *et al.* 1991). The association of sexual behaviour with HPV status has not yet been adequately defined.

4.9   Evidence for non-sexual transmission

There is more direct evidence implicating possible non-sexual transmission. HPV 16/18 DNA sequences have been demonstrated in nasopharyngeal aspirates from neonates, laryngeal tissue from infants, and cytological samples from virgins (Ley *et al.* 1991; Sedlacek *et al.* 1989; Young *et al.* (unpublished)) (Table 4.3). There are other possible routes of infection. HPV 16/18 DNA sequences have been isolated from normal buccal mucosa in 44 per cent and 23 per cent of healthy young adults (Jalal *et al.* 1992; Kellokoski *et al.* 1992). The conclusion seems inescapable that some but not all cervical HPV infection is acquired by means other than sexual intercourse.

4.10   Role of HPV testing in clinical practice

One reviewer has compared the possible use of HPV testing as a primary screening procedure to 'screening for hypertension by asking about salt

Table 4.3 Evidence for non-sexual transmission

		Site	Detection method	Number (%) HPV positive
Infants	Birmingham *n* = 70	Larynx	PCR	19 (27%)
	USA *n* = 45	Nasopharyngeal aspirates	SB	15 (33%)
Virgins	Birmingham *n* = 17	Cervix	PCR	12 (64%)
	USA *n* = 15	Vulva	PCR	3 (20%)

consumption, without measuring blood pressure' (Beral and Day 1992). Inappropriate as a primary screening procedure, the highly significant association between HPV status and CIN has persuaded some that HPV status might usefully be exploited as an adjunct to cytological examination (Cuzick *et al.* 1992; Bavin *et al.* 1992).

Nuova *et al.* (1992) used HPV testing to tackle a not uncommon clinical dilemma—the woman found to have no colposcopic abnormality after referral for investigation of cytological abnormality. HPV testing at the time of colposcopic assessment correctly predicted 78 per cent of those who were subsequently diagnosed as having CIN within the next 12 months. But the simpler and cheaper expedient of repeat cytological testing at the time of the next colposcopic examination, however, provided an even better prediction (92 per cent) of the eventual histological diagnosis of CIN. A significant association does not a sensitive screening test make and it seems unlikely in the light of current knowledge that HPV testing will increase the efficiency of cytological examination (see also Chapter 3).

4.11 Temporal trends in prevalence of HPV infections

Routinely collected surveillance data on sexually transmitted disease are often quoted as showing a substantial increase in the incidence of genital warts (Department of Health 1990). The true magnitude of this increase is uncertain given that these statistics count clinical consultations and not patients, and are likely to be confounded by temporal trends in self-reporting and service utilization. In any event, the relevance of the observation to cervical cancer is not clear. Although associated with CIN, no convincing evidence has been adduced linking a history of exposure to genital warts with invasive disease (Muñoz and Bosch 1992). This is perhaps not surprising, given that genital warts are thought to be associated with 'low-risk' HPV types. The major impact of the increase in the reported number of women with genital warts may have been the additional burden placed on the colposcopy services arising from the investigation and treatment of the minor cytological abnormalities associated with these lesions.

The interpretation of temporal trends in the prevalence of subclinical disease is made difficult by the changes in diagnostic awareness. A review of 995 colposcopically directed punch biopsies revealed a significant increase in the reporting of histological evidence of HPV infection over a ten-year period but when the material was independently re-examined by one pathologist no significant increase in the prevalence of HPV was found (Byrne *et al.* 1986). Longitudinal observations on sufficient numbers of subjects have not yet been made and therefore reliable estimates of the incidence of subclinical infection are not yet widely available. The most robust estimate of the incidence of cytologically defined subclinical infection has been provided by the rescreening of a cohort of Finnish women. When the observed incidence in this cohort was combined with the age-specific prevalence of cytological HPV infection in older age groups, the cumulative lifetime risk of developing subclinical infection was found to be 79 per cent (Syrjänen *et al.* 1990).

It has only been possible to examine temporal trends in the prevalence of latent HPV infection by using archival material. These suggest that there has been little change in the prevalence of HPV DNA sequences in cytological material over the period 1972–87 or in the prevalence of HPV DNA in a sample of cervical cancers which were removed over a fifty-year period extending from 1922 (Rakoczy *et al.* 1990; Thompson *et al.* 1992). These cross-sectional comparisons suggest that we are not describing a new phenomenon. It would be interesting to determine if the well-documented cohort trends in the incidence of cervical carcinoma reflect changes in the prevalence of HPV infection.

4.12   Extragenital HPV infection

'High risk' HPV DNA sequences have been detected at a number of extragenital sites. Some investigators have sampled only malignant tissue (Fig. 4.3) (Yousem *et al.* 1992; Chang *et al.* 1990; Shindoh *et al.* 1992; Huang *et al.* 1992; Perez-Ayala *et al.* 1990). Others report the prevalence of HPV DNA in malignant tissue and biopsy specimens removed from normal controls (Fig. 4.4) (Benamouzig *et al.* 1992; Rotola *et al.* 1992; Anwar *et al.* 1992, 1993; Snijders *et al.* 1992). Only one formal case-control study of the etiological role of HPV in the genesis of extragenital neoplasia has been reported. This demonstrated a significant association with the finding of HPV 6 DNA sequences and oral cancer (odds ratio = 2.9, 95 per cent CI 1.1, 7.3) and a non-significant relationship with the detection of HPV 16 (odds ratio = 6.7 95 per cent CI 0.7, 52.2) (Maden *et al.* 1992). Some believe that the non-specific tissue tropism of HPV undermines the case for an etiological role in cervical neoplasia. Tobacco consumption, however, has also been linked to squamous neoplasia at different sites and an interaction with HPV exposure has been suggested. Although such a relationship is conceivable in cervical neoplasia, it seems less plausible for cancers at other sites in the aerodigestive tract where the risks attributable to smoking are much higher. Further case-control studies examining the role of HPV in squamous neoplasia at other sites are urgently needed.

4.13   The future

Two problems face those who attempt to more precisely determine the association between the development of cervical neoplasia and the acqui-

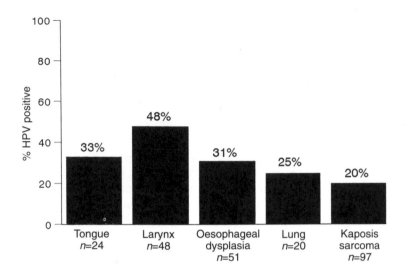

Fig. 4.3 Distribution of HPV 16, 18, 33, or 35 DNA sequences in extragenital neoplastic tissue.

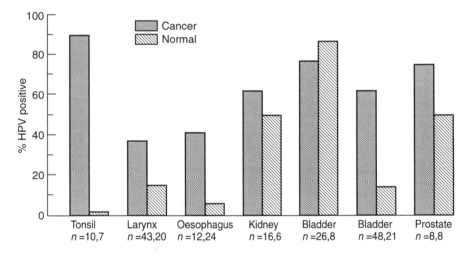

Fig. 4.4 Distribution of HPV 16, 18, 33, or 35 DNA sequences in extragenital neoplastic and normal tissue.

sition of HPV infection: first, the need to generate a series of longitudinal observations on a cohort of women at risk of the disease; and second, to develop a robust methodology able to detect the presence of HPV DNA sequences in the small volumes of DNA which would be provided by serial cytological samples.

When PCR technology was first used to detect the presence of HPV DNA sequences in cytologically normal smears, the prevalence of infection was found to be substantially greater than that previously predicted using other techniques.

The implications of these findings were considerable. The high prevalence of HPV DNA in normal epithelium was considered to make an etiological role for this virus in the genesis of cervical neoplasia less likely. Subsequent investigations using this technique suggested that HPV could not only be detected in the genital tract of those who had yet to embark on sexual activity but also at a number of extragenital sites. These findings threatened a long-cherished hypothesis. The first published indication that the PCR technology was not as robust as had previously been hoped came with the retraction of a report by Tidy *et al.* (1989) describing a subtype of HPV 16 (HPV 16B) which they believed to be a variant of HPV 16 closely associated with cervical neoplasia. Subsequent reports drew attention to the problems of accidental sample cross-contamination or PCR product carry-over and argued that use of the PCR necessitated stringent laboratory procedures. Contemporaneous with these reports there emerged a series of prevalence studies which provided widely differing estimates of the prevalence of genital HPV infection (Young *et al.* 1992). Perhaps inevitably those studies which reported a high prevalence were considered methodologically unsound whereas those 'epidemiologically friendly' studies which reported a low prevalence were considered more acceptable and thought to result from a more fastidious methodology. That these studies were undertaken in very different and often poorly characterized populations was noted but its relevance perhaps not fully appreciated by a discomforted, confused, and now somewhat defensive cadre of molecular biologists.

The PCR has recently enjoyed something of a cautious renaissance. It is clear, however, that possible methodological differences in the application of this technique still need to be carefully considered. The first consideration relates to the choice of primers. The initial studies used type-specific HPV primers directed at the early region of the viral genome. This approach was subsequently modified in an attempt to prevent contamination by using primers which flanked the HPV cloning site. More recently, consensus primers directed at highly conserved regions of the HPV genome have been used. These consensus primers are not, however, type-specific. The extent to which the use of different primers may confound comparisons of the prevalence of HPV 16 DNA in different populations has only recently been formally examined. We have shown that the prevalence of HPV 16 in abnormal cervical smears did not vary with the use of primers directed at early or late regions of the viral genome but that the prevalence in normal smears was substantially less when primers directed at the early region were used (Tierney *et al.* 1993). Differential misclassification following the use of certain primers will confound case-control comparisons.

The interpretation of a positive PCR remains a largely unaddressed issue. When a technique can detect as little as one copy of the genome per 10 cells (DeBritton *et al.* 1993), the biological importance of detecting such small amounts of DNA needs to be considered. Some investigators have already capitulated and recommended the use of less sensitive techniques when attempting to demonstrate case-control differences in the prevalence of HPV DNA. A less nihilistic approach would include combining the sensitivity of PCR with the cellular localization afforded by *in situ* hybridization in order to further elucidate the biological and clinical importance of a positive results. Also, a more robust quantitation of the PCR than has been previously described might be expected to explain or elucidate the somewhat disconcerting finding of HPV 16 DNA sequences in a wide variety of normal and abnormal epithelia. Resolution of these methodological uncertainties is necessary if we are to derive useful information from the large-scale epidemiological inquiries which are already underway.

References

Anwar, K., Naiki, H., Makakuki, K., and Inuzuka, M. (1992). High frequency of human papillomavirus infection in carcinoma of the urinary bladder. *Cancer*, **70**, 1967–73.

Anwar, K., Nakakuki, K., Naiki, H., and Inuzuka, M. (1993). RAs gene mutations and HPV infection are common in human laryngeal carcinoma. *International Journal of Cancer*, **53**, 22–8.

Azocar, J., Abad, S. M. J., Acosta, H., Hernandez, R., Gallegos, M., Pifano, E. *et al.* (1990). Prevalence of cervical dysplasia and HPV infection according to sexual behaviour. *International Journal of Cancer*, **45**, 622–5

Bavin, P. J., Giles, J. A., Hudson, E., Williams, D., Crow, J., Griffiths, P. *et al.* (1992). Comparison of cervical cytology and the polymerase chain reaction for HPV 16 to identify women with cervical disease in a general practice population. *Journal of Medical Virology*, **37**, 8–12.

Benamouzig, R., Pigot, F., Quiroga, G., Validire, P., Chaussade, S., Catalan, F. *et al.* (1992). Human papillomavirus infection in esophageal squamous-cell carcinoma in western countries. *International Journal of Cancer*, **50**, 549–52.

Beral, V. and Day, N. E. (1992). Screening for cervical cancer: is there a place for incorporating tests for the human papillomavirus? In *The epidemiology of cervical cancer and human papillomavirus* (eds. N. Munoz, F. X. Bosch, K. V. Shah and A. Meheus). IARC, Lyon.

Burkett, B. J., Peterson, C. M., Birch, L. M., Brennan, C., Nuckols, M. L., Ward, B. E. *et al.* (1992). The relationship between contraceptives, sexual practices, and cervical human papillomavirus infection among a college population. *Journal of Clinical Epidemiology*, **45**, 1295–302.

Byrne, P., Woodman, C. B. J., Meanwell, C. A., and Jordan, J. A. (1986). Changing awareness of human papillomavirus infection. *Lancet*, **1**, 205.

Campion, M. J., McCance, D. J., Cuzick, J., and Singer, A. (1986). Progressive potential of mild cervical atypia: prospective cytological, colposcopic, and virological study. *Lancet*, **2**, 237–40.

Chang, F., Syrjanen, S., Shen, Q., Ji, H., and Syrjanen, K. (1990). Human papillomavirus (HPV) DNA in esophageal precancer lesions and squamous cell carcinomas from China. *International Journal of Cancer*, **45**, 21–5.

Cuzick, J., Terry, G., Ho, L., Hollingworth, T., and Anderson, M. (1992). Human papillomavirus type 16 DNA in cervical smears as predictor of high-grade cervical cancer. *Lancet*, **339**, 959–60.

De Villiers, E-M., Wagner, D., Schneider, A., Wesch, H., Munz, F., Miklaw, H. et al. (1992). Human Papillomavirus DNA in women without and with cytological abnormalities: results of a 5-year follow-up study. *Gynecologic Oncology*, **44**, 33–9.

DeBritton, R. C., Hildesheim, A., De Lao, S. L., Brinton, L. A., Sathya, P., and Reeves, W. C. (1993). Human papillomaviruses and other influences on survival from cervical cancer in Panama. *Obstetrics & Gynecology*, **81**, 19–24.

Department of Health SM14B. New cases seen at NHS genito-urinary medicine clinics in England: 1990 Annual and December Quarter Figures.

Guerrero, E., Daniel, R. W., Bosch, F. X., Castellsague, X., Munoz, N., Gili, M. et al. (1992). Comparison of virapap, southern hybridization, and polymerase chain reaction methods for human papillomavirus identification in an epidemiological investigation of cervical cancer. *Journal of Clinical Microbiology*, **30**, 2951–9.

Hennekens, C. H. and Buring, J. E. (1987). Case-control studies. In *Epidemiology in Medicine* (ed. S. L. M. Mayrent), pp. 132–52. Little, Brown and Co., Boston/Toronto.

Higgins, G. D., Davy, M., Roder, D., Uzelin, D. M., Phillips, G. E., and Burrell, C. J. (1991). Increased age and mortality associated with cervical carcinomas negative for human papillomavirus RNA. *Lancet*, **338**, 910–13.

Hildesheim, A., Mann, V., Brinton, L. A., Szklo, M., Reeves, W. C., and Rawls, W. E. (1991). Herpes simplex virus type 2: A possible interaction with human papillomavirus types 16/18 in the development of invasive cervical cancer. *International Journal of Cancer*, **49**, 335–40.

Huang, Y. Q., Li, J. J., Rush, M. G., Poiesz, B. J., Nicolaides, A., Jacobson, M. et al. (1992). HPV-16-related DNA sequences in Kaposi's sarcoma. *Lancet*, **339**, 515–18.

Jalal, H., Snaders, C. M., Prime, S. S., Scully, C., and Maitland, N. J. (1992). Detection of human papillomavirus type 16 DNA in oral squames from normal young adults. *Journal of Oral Pathol. Medicine.*, **21**, 465–70.

Kellokoski, J. K., Syrjanen, S. M., Chang, F., Yliskoski, M., and Syrjanen, K. J. (1992). Southern blot hybridization and PCR in detection of oral human papillomavirus (HPV) infections in women with genital HPV infections. *Journal of Oral Pathol. Medicine*, **21**, 459–64.

Kiviat, N. B., Koutsky, L. A., Paavonen, J. A., Galloway, D. A., Critchlow, C. W., Beckmann, A. M. et al. (1989). Prevalence of genital papillomavirus infection among women attending a college student health clinic or a sexually transmitted disease clinic. *Journal of Infectious Diseases*, **159**, 293–302.

Kjaer, S. K., Engholm, G., Teisen, C., Augaard, B. J., Lynge, E., Christensen, R. B. et al. (1992). Risk factors for cervical human papillomavirus and herpes simplex virus infections in Greenland and Denmark: a population based study. *American Journal of Epidemiology*, **131**, 669–82.

Koutsky, L. A., Holmes, K. K., Critchlow, S. W., Stevens, C. E., Paavonen, J., Beckmann, A. M. *et al.* (1992). A cohort study of the risk of cervical intra-epithelial neoplasia grade 2 or 3 in relation to papillomavirus infection. *New England Journal of Medicine*, **327**, 1272–8.

Ley, C., Bauer, H. M., Reingold, A., Schiffman, M. H., Chambers, J. C., Tashiro, C. J. *et al.* (1991). Determinants of genital human papillomavirus infection in young women. *Journal of the National Cancer Institute*, **83**, 997–1003.

Maden, C., Beckmann, A. M., Thomas, D. B., McKnight, B., Sherman, K., Ashley, J. *et al.* (1992). Human papillomaviruses, herpes simplex viruses, and the risk of oral cancer in men. *American Journal of Epidemiology*, **135**, 1093–102.

Meanwell, C. A., Blackledge, G., Cox, M. F., and Maitland, N. J. (1987). HPV 16 DNA in normal and malignant cervical epithelium: implications for the aetiology and behaviour of cervical neoplasia. *Lancet*, **I**, 703–7.

Morrison, E. A. B., Ho, G. Y. F., Vermund, S. H., Goldberg, G. L., Kadish, A. S., Kelley, K. F. *et al.* (1991). Human papillomavirus infection and other risk factors for cervical neoplasia: a case-control study. *International Journal of Cancer*, **49**, 6–13.

Moscicki, A., Palefsky, J., Gonzales, J., and Schoolnik, G. K. (1990). Human papillomavirus infection in sexually active adolescent females: prevalence and risk factors. *Pediatric Research*, **28**, 507–13.

Mugica-van Herckenrode, C., Malcolm, A. D. B., and Coleman, D. V. (1992). Prevalence of human papillomavirus (HPV) infection in Basque country women using slot-blot hybridization: a survey of women at low risk of developing cervical cancer. *International Journal of Cancer*, **51**, 581–6.

Muñoz, N., Bosch, F. X., De Sanjose, S., Tafur, L., Izarzugaza, I., Gili, M. *et al.* (1992). The causal link between human papillomavirus and invasive cervical cancer: a population-based case-control study in Columbia and Spain. *International Journal of Cancer*, **52**, 743–9.

Muñoz, N. and Bosch, F. X. (1992). HPV and cervical neoplasia: Review of case-control and cohort studies. In *The epidemiology of cervical cancer and human papillomavirus* (eds. N. Muñoz, F. X. Bosch, K. V. Shah, and A. Meheus). International Agency for Research on Cancer (IARC), Lyon.

Murthy, N. S., Sehgal, A., Satyanarayana, L., Das, D. K., Singh, V., Das, B. C. *et al.* (1990). Risk factors related to biological behaviour of precancerous lesions of the uterine cervix. *British Journal of Cancer*, **61**, 732–6.

Nuovo, G. J., Moritz, J., Walsh, L. L., Macconnell, P., and Koulos, J. (1992). Predictive value of human papillomavirus DNA detection by filter hybridization and polymerase chain reaction in women with negative results of colposcopic examination. *American Journal of Clinical Pathology*, **98**, 489–92.

Peng, H., Liu, S., Mann, V., Rohan, T., and Rawls, W. (1991). Human papillomavirus types 16 and 33, herpes simplex virus type 2 and other risk factors for cervical cancer in Sichuan province, China. *International Journal of Cancer*, **47**, 711–16.

Perez-Ayala, M., Ruiz-Cabello, F., Esteban, F., Concha, A., Redondo, M., Oliva, M. R. *et al.* (1990). Presence of HPV 16 sequences in laryngeal carcinomas. *International Journal of Cancer*, **46**, 8–11.

Rakoczy, P., Sterett, G., Kulski, J., Whitaker, D., Hutchinson, L., Mackenzie, J. *et al.* (1990). Time trends in the prevalence of human papillomavirus infections in archival Papanicolaou smears: analysis by cytology, DNA hybridization, and polymerase chain reaction. *Journal of Medical Virology*, **32**, 10–17.

Reeves, W. C., Brinton, L. A., Garcia, M., Brenes, M. M., Herrero, R., Gaitan, E. *et al.* (1989). Human papillomavirus infection and cervical cancer in Latin America. *New England Journal of Medicine*, **320**, 1437–41.

Riou, G., Favre, M., Jeannel, D., Bourhis, J., LeDoussal, V., and Orth, G. (1990). Association between poor prognosis in early-stage invasive cervical carcinomas and non-detection of HPV DNA. *Lancet*, **335**, 1171–4.

Rogentine, G. N., Trapani, R. J., Yankee, R. A. and Henderson, E. S. (1973). HL-A antigens and acute lymphocytic leukaemia: the nature of the HL-A2 association. *Tissue Antigens*, **3**, 470.

Rohan, T., Mann, V., McLaughlin, J., Harnish, D. G., Yu, H., Smith, D. *et al.* (1991). PCR-Detected genital papillomavirus infection: prevalence and association with risk factors for cervical cancer. *International Journal of Cancer*, **49**, 856–60.

Rosenfeld, W. D., Vermund, S. H., Wentz, S. J., and Burk, R. D. (1989). High prevalence rate of human papillomavirus infection and association with abnormal Papanicolaou smears in sexually active adolescents. *American Journal of Diseases in Children*, **143**, 1443–7.

Rotola, A., Monini, P., Di Luca, D., Savioli, A., Simone, R., Secchiero, P. *et al.* (1992). Presence and physical state of HPV DNA in prostate and urinary-tract tissues. *International Journal of Cancer*, **52**, 359–65.

Schmauz, R., Okong, P., De Villiers, E-M., Dennin, R., Brade, L., Lwanga, S. K. *et al.* (1989). Multiple infections in cases of cervical cancer from a high-incidence area in tropical Africa. *International Journal of Cancer*, **43**, 805–9.

Sedlacek, T. V., Lindheim, S., Eder, C., Hasty, L., Woodland, M., Ludomirsky, A. *et al.* (1989). Mechanism for human papillomavirus transmission at birth. *American Journal of Obstetrics and Gynecology*, **161**, 55–9.

Shindoh, M., Sawada, Y., Kohgo, T., Amemiya, A., and Fujinaga, K. (1992). Detection of human papillomavirus DNA sequences in tongue squamous-cell carcinoma utilizing the polymerase chain reaction method. *International Journal of Cancer*, **50**, 167–71.

Snijders, P. J. F., Cromme, F. V., Van Den Brule, A. J. C., Schrijnemakers, H. F. J., Snow, G. B., Meijer, C. J. L. M. *et al.* (1992). Prevalence and expression of human papillomavirus in tonsillar carcinomas, indicating a possible viral etiology. *International Journal of Cancer*, **51**, 845–50.

Syrjanen, K., Hakama, M., Saarikoski, S., Vayrynen, M., Yliskoski, M., Syrjanen, S. *et al.* (1990). Prevalence, incidence, and estimated life-time risk of cervical human papillomavirus infections in a nonselected Finnish female population. *Sexually Transmitted Diseases*, **17**, 15–19.

Ter Meulen, J., Eberhardt, H. C., Luande, J., Mgaya, H. N., Chang-Claude, J., Mtiro, H. *et al.* (1992). Human papillomavirus (HPV) infection, HIV infection and cervical cancer in Tanzania, East Africa. *International Journal of Cancer*, **51**, 515–21.

Thompson, C. H., Rose, B. R., and Cossart, Y. E. (1992). Detection of HPV DNA in archival specimens of cervical cancer using in situ hybridization and the polymerase chain reaction. *Journal of Medical Virology*, **36**, 54–9.

Tidy, J. A., Parry, G. C. N., Ward, P. *et al.* (1989). High rate of human papillomavirus type 16 infection in cytologically normal cervices. *Lancet*, **i**, 434.

Tierney, R., Ellis, J., Winter, H., Kaureshi, H., Wilson, S., Woodman, C. B. J. *et al.* (1993). PCR for the detection of cervical HPV 16 infection: the need for standardisation. *International Journal of Cancer*, in press.

Van Doornum, G. J. J., Hooykaas, C., Juffermans, L. H. J., Van Der Lans, S. M. G. A., Van Der Linden, M. M. D., Coutinho, R. A. *et al.* (1992). Prevalence of human papillomavirus infections among heterosexual men and women with multiple sexual partners. *Journal of Medical Virology*, **37**, 13–21.

Young, L. S., Tierney, R. J., Ellis, J. R. M., Winter, H., and Woodman, C. B. J. (1992). PCR for the detection of genital human papillomavirus infection: a mixed blessing. *Annals of Medicine*, **24**, 215–19.

Young, L. S., Johnson, M., Blomfield, P., and Woodman, C. B. J. Prevalence of HPV 16 DNA sequences in laryngeal tissue taken from infants with SIDS and in cytological samples taken from virgins (unpublished data).

Yousem, S. A., Ohori, N. P., and Sonmez-Alpan, E. (1992). Occurrence of human papillomavirus DNA in primary lung neoplasms. *Cancer*, **69**, 693–7.

5 Mechanisms of transformation by HPV

KAREN H. VOUSDEN

5.1 Introduction

Cervical carcinoma has long been recognized as a sexually transmitted disease and, as described in Chapter 4, there is now extremely convincing epidemiological evidence that infection with certain types of genital human papillomaviruses (HPVs), known as the high-risk HPVs, contribute to the development of this cancer. The identification of some HPV types as oncogenic viruses has not solely been the result of epidemiological studies, however, and some of the most compelling evidence implicating the malignant potential of these viruses has been gathered from the study of *in vitro* transformation mediated by HPV DNA. Although the ability to efficiently transform cells in culture is, by itself, no safe indication that a virus has malignant potential *in vivo* (as illustrated by the adenoviruses), the identification and analysis of HPV-encoded oncogenes has reinforced the hypothesis that HPV infection plays a causative role in the development of most cervical cancers. More recently, an understanding of how the virally encoded oncoproteins function is paving the path towards the development of better prognostic and diagnostic tests, as well as prophylactic or therapeutic drugs and vaccines.

5.2 Transformation by HPVs

The initial step in understanding the mechanisms by which the high-risk HPV types function in cervical cell transformation was the detection of transforming and immortalizing activities following introduction of the viral DNA into cultured cells, indicating that the viruses themselves encode proteins which can participate in malignant transformation. Analysis of the small viral genome rapidly led to the identification of viral genes which, when expressed in suitable recipient cells, could participate in at least one step of malignant transformation (Vousden 1991b). Initial studies were carried out in rodent cells, using primary cells to analyse immortalizing activity of transfected genes or established cell lines in which transformation to phenotypes such as anchorage independence, loss of growth factor dependence, or tumourigenicity can be assayed (Vousden 1991a). Using such assays both the immortalizing and transforming activities detected in full-length HPV 16 or 18 DNA were shown to be principally due to expression of the E7 open reading frame (ORF), although more recent studies have shown that weaker activities can also be assigned to E6 and E5. As described in Chapter 2, at least some of the HPV DNA often becomes integrated into the host genome during the development of many cervical cancers, resulting in the loss or lack of expression of much of the viral genome. The identification of the E6 and E7 ORFs in transformation assays was of particular interest since these are the only two viral genes which are consistenly maintained and expressed in cervical cancers and are therefore excellent candidates for genes which are likely to play a role in both the development and maintenance of these malignancies.

Rodent cells, unlike human cells, are easily transformed and immortalized and the importance of E6 and E7 was greatly strengthened by subsequent studies using primary human genital epithelial cells. Like most primary cells taken from the animal, human epithelial cells have only a finite lifespan, after which they irreversibly stop proliferating. Simultaneous expression of both E6 and E7 extends this lifespan and since some of these cells have been dividing in culture for five or more years they can be considered immortal. In these human cells cooperation between E6 and E7 is necessary for efficient immortalization (Hawley-Nelson *et al.* 1989; Münger *et al.* 1989). Interestingly, the immortalized human cells show abnormal differentiation patterns in organotypic culture conditions and give rise to an epithelium which very closely resembles the pre-neoplastic cervical lesion, cervical intra-epithelial neoplasia (Hudson *et al.* 1990). The ability of HPV proteins to allow unscheduled proliferation of human genital epithelial cells is potentially important in contributing to malignant development, but the additional defect in normal differentiation of these cells provides some of the strongest experimental evidence that HPV infection directly results in the genesis of a pre-cancerous condition.

5.3   Activities of high- and low-risk viruses

The division of genital HPV types into high and low risk depending on the frequency with which they appear in cervical cancers prompted a comparison of the *in vitro* immortalizing and transforming activities of the E6 and E7 proteins encoded by these two groups of viruses. In all the assays examined, in both rodent and human cells, E6 and E7 encoded by low-risk viruses (such as HPV6 or HPV11) showed a dramatically lower activity than those encoded by high-risk viruses (such as HPV16 or 18). This correlation between *in vivo* and *in vitro* activities again supports a role for E6 and E7 in the development of HPV-associated cancers. These studies did indicate, however, that all E6 and E7 proteins showed some potential to perform in these assays, but that the proteins encoded by the high-risk viruses function with a much higher efficiency. This was particularly clearly illustrated by studies which showed that combinations of E6 and E7 from high- and low-risk viruses had immortalizing activities intermediate between those obtained using either both high- or both low-risk virus-encoded proteins (Halbert *et al.* 1992). It therefore appears that both the high- and low-risk genital HPV-encoded E6 and E7 proteins show some ability to disrupt the normal control of cell growth and contribute to cell transformation. This may be a reflection of the *in vivo* activities of these viruses, where infection with even the low-risk HPV types typically results in marked hyperproliferation and the appearance of benign condylomatous lesions.

5.4   E6 and E7 interaction with cell proteins

At least some of the mechanisms by which the HPV oncoproteins function have been identified by virtue of their similarity with the oncoproteins encoded by other DNA viruses such as adenovirus and simian virus 40 (SV40) (Fig. 5.1) (Green 1989). The transforming proteins encoded by all three groups of viruses interact with the same cell proteins, which have subsequently been shown to be important regulators of cell growth. It has been suggested that this remarkable similarity between otherwise unrelated viruses is a reflection of the necessity to disrupt the control of cell growth and sustain proliferation in a cell population which would normally cease division. The natural role of the viral transforming proteins would therefore be the induction or maintenance of a cell environment in which viral replication can take place. These small viruses rely heavily on host-encoded components for successful proliferation, and induction of cellular replication ensures that the necessary factors for viral replication are being synthesized. The ability of the viral proteins to interfere with the factors governing the regulation of cell growth may contribute to malignant progression, for example following a failure in the normal viral infective cycle.

5.5   Cell cycle regulation

Cell proliferation proceeds by an ordered and complex series of events which constitute the cell cycle (Fig. 5.2). Actively dividing cells pass through distinct stages of DNA synthesis (S-phase) and mitotic division (M-phase) and these periods of obvious activity are separated by gaps (G1 and G2),

HPV

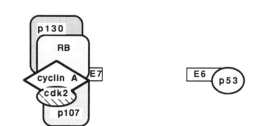

Adenovirus

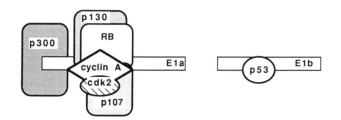

SV40

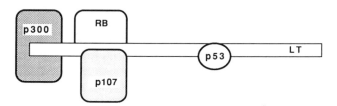

Fig. 5.1 HPV, adenovirus, and SV40 encode transforming proteins which form complexes with a similar group of cellular proteins. The LT:p300 association shown is based on indirect evidence. All the known interactions have been shown simultaneously for convenience rather than to imply the formation of a complex containing all the indicated proteins.

during which checks on the fidelity of division and preparation of the next phase take place. Control of the cell cycle is enormously complex, involving many interconnecting pathways of regulation. Central to this control are a family of kinases, known as cyclin-dependent kinases (Pines and Hunter 1991), which play a pivotal role in controlling progress into both S and M phase. Active forms of these enzymes consist of a catalytic subunit, encoded by the *cdk* gene family, associated with a regulatory subunit from the family of proteins called cyclins and the tightly controlled activity of these kinases through the cell cycle appears to be critical for

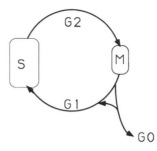

Fig. 5.2 A typical eukaryotic cell cycle. DNA synthesis (S phase) and mitotic division (M phase) are separated by two gaps (G1 and G2). Cells may leave the active cell cycle by entering a poorly defined phase, G0.

ordered progression through cell division. Increasing numbers of cdks and cyclins are being identified and the number of potential variants of these enzymes is even further increased by the ability of the two subunits to associate in various combinations (Xiong and Beach 1991).

Throughout normal proliferation a series of checkpoints and feedback controls operate to monitor accuracy and completion of various stages of the cell cycle. These checkpoints are extremely important and failure to satisfy conditions for progression results in arrest and possible exit from the cell cycle (Murray 1992). If nutrient or growth factor levels become inadequate for the maintenance of growth, for example, the cell may enter quiescence (G0), a reversible state from which the cell can re-enter the cycle if conditions improve. Irreversible exit from the cell cycle also occurs as cells follow pathways of differentiation, senescence, or programmed death known as apoptosis.

Perturbations of any of the normal controls of cell proliferation potentially contribute to malignant conversion, either by gain of inappropriate positive signals or loss of controlling negative signals. The identification of the targets of HPV oncoproteins as some of the components involved in cell cycle regulation has allowed a fascinating insight into how the viral proteins function.

5.6   E7 interactions with Rb, a tumour suppressor gene product

Several cell proteins have now been shown to form complexes with E7 (Fig. 5.1) and the interaction between E7 and the protein encoded by the retinoblastoma gene, *Rb-1*, is one of the best understood. The *Rb-1* gene belongs to a growing family of tumour suppressor genes which characteristically suffer a loss of function by mutation in both alleles during cancer development (Marshall 1991). The products of such genes would be expected to be involved in preventing or delaying progress through the cell cycle and therefore act as inhibitors or negative regulators of cell growth. Loss of this control by inactivation of the tumour suppressor gene product would be anticipated to contribute to malignant development. The genetic basis for the development of retinoblastoma was originally proposed by Knudson (1971), based on the observation that many of these childhood tumours occur in a familial form. Hereditary retinoblastomas often present as multiple tumours in both eyes, and patients who inherit this syndrome show a predisposition to develop other malignancies later in life. Retinoblastoma may also occur in a sporadic form, however, which usually presents as a single, unilateral tumour. Knudson postulated that this would be characteristic of a cancer in which two independent genetic events play an important role, and subsequent studies have shown these to be mutations within the two alleles of the retinoblastoma gene, *Rb-1*, resulting in the loss of functional Rb protein. Hereditary predisposition to cancer is seen in patients who inherit a mutation in one allele of the tumour suppressor gene, in this case *Rb-1*, and therefore require only a single somatic event to inactivate the remaining allele and suffer complete loss of tumour suppressor protein function. In the sporadic cancers, two independent genetic events to inactivate both alleles are necessary and these cancers are concomitantly less common. Subsequent molecular analyses have shown that mutations affecting *Rb-1* can be identified in several other types of human cancer, indicating that the contribution of Rb to the control of malignant development is not restricted to retinoblastoma cells. The loss of Rb function in the development of cancers other than retinoblastomas is particularly interesting when considering HPV associated cervical cancers, where inactivation of Rb appears to occur as a result of the interaction with the virally encoded E7 protein, rather than mutation within the *Rb-1* gene itself.

5.7 Functions of Rb

The function of Rb appears to be related to its ability to complex and control the activity of other cell proteins, such as E2F and *myc*, which themselves function as transcription factors (Hamel *et al.* 1992a). Control of transcription is thought to be a key mechanism by which progress through the cell cycle is regulated (McKinney and Heintz 1991) and there is evidence that E2F is involved in controlling transcription of several genes important for entry into the cycle and progress through G1 into S phase. Since the association between E2F and Rb prevents transcriptional activation by E2F (and may even actively repress transcription from

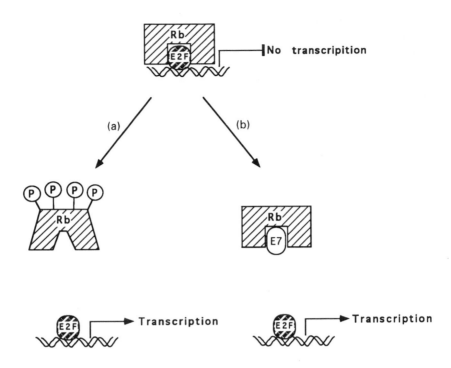

Fig. 5.3 Possible mechanisms to overcome negative growth regulation by Rb. The complex between E2F and Rb is unable to direct transcription from E2F responsive promotors. (a) Following cell cycle regulated phosporylation by a cyclin-dependent kinase, the complex dissociates and subsequent expression of other cellular genes results in entry into DNA synthesis. Note that this sequence of events is precipitated by the activation of the appropriate cyclin-dependent kinase. (b) The normal regulation of E2F responsive genes can be disrupted following association between E7 and unphosphorylated Rb and disruption of the Rb/E2F complex.

E2F-responsive elements (Dalton 1992; Hamel *et al.* 1992b; Weintraub *et al.* 1992)), the interaction enables Rb to participate in the control of cell proliferation by preventing expression of E2F-regulated genes. In a normal cell the Rb protein is sequentially phosphorylated throughout the cell cycle and this is likely to be one of the mechanisms by which Rb function is controlled, although additional mechanisms which regulate function also exist (Goodrich *et al.* 1991). The exciting observation that Rb is phosphorylated by a member of the cyclin-dependent kinases, combined with evidence that expression of certain cyclins can overcome the growth-suppressing function of Rb (Hinds *et al.* 1992), suggests that cdks may regulate advance through the cell cycle, at least in part by controlling Rb function. Phosphorylated forms of Rb lose the ability to complex with

E2F and the subsequent release of active E2F could result in transcription of the genes necessary for further cell cycle progression (Fig. 5.3). This simple model of Rb function is complicated somewhat by the observation that Rb:E2F complex persists well into S phase, past the point where the first round of Rb phosphorylation is detected, and it is possible that the persistence of this Rb complex is to actively repress transcription of genes such as *myc* (Schwartz *et al.* 1993). Although interaction with E2F is important, Rb also functions through E2F-independent mechanisms (Kim *et al.* 1992) and recent evidence suggests that in addition to its role in cell cycle progression, active Rb is necessary for terminal differentiation (Gu *et al.* 1993). The interaction between E7 and Rb disrupts the association with E2F (Chellappan *et al.* 1992) and E7 expression might therefore lead to the inappropriate transcription of E2F-responsive genes and release of the normal blocks on progress through the cell cycle (Fig. 5.3). This is supported by the observations that E7 expression can activate transcription through E2F-responsive elements (Phelps *et al.* 1991) and identification of E7 functions at G0 and G1, precisely those stages of the cell cycle predicted to be regulated by E2F-responsive gene products (Sato *et al.* 1989; Banks *et al.* 1990a).

5.8   The Rb-related protein, p107

Rb has recently been shown to be one of a family of proteins which have the ability to complex transcription factors such as E2F. Temporal differences in the formation of complexes between E2F and the Rb protein family throughout the cell cycle, resulting in a complex pattern of expression of the active form of E2F, almost certainly contribute to the strict regulation of E2F-responsive genes. p107, the best characterized of the Rb-related proteins, forms a complex with E2F at least twice, once during early G1 and again during S phase and therefore appears to be involved in E2F regulation at more than one stage of the cell cycle (Nevins 1992). Although p107 probably negatively regulates E2F in a manner similar to Rb, the association between p107 and E2F may provide functions in addition to the regulation of E2F transcriptional control. Both G1 and S phase forms of the p107:E2F complex can also contain a member of the cdk family; cdk2 with cyclin E at G1 and cdk2 with cyclin A during S phase although a G1 complex containing only E2F and p107 has also been detected (Schwartz *et al.* 1993). Since E2F has a specific DNA binding activity, these complexes could play a role in specifically targeting the kinases to other DNA bound proteins. Recent studies have shown that E7 also forms a complex with p107 (Fig. 5.1) (Dyson *et al.* 1992; Davies *et al.* 1993) and potentially E7 could interfere with all these regulatory interactions.

5.9   Association of E7 with a cyclin-dependent kinase

Most of the activities of E7 which have been described so far appear to relate to the ability of E7 to allow progression through the early stages of the cell cycle into DNA synthesis. There are, however, also important cell cycle control points after S phase and there is some evidence that E7 can participate in progress through G2 into mitosis (Vousden and Jat 1989). The basis of such an E7 function is much less well understood, but recent studies have identified one activity of E7 that might be important at this stage of the cell cycle. E7 has been shown to associate with a cyclin-dependent kinase activity by binding cyclin A and cdk2 (Fig. 5.1) (Tommasino *et al.* 1993). Since these kinases play such an important role in regulating progress through the cell cycle, any alteration of their normal function could disrupt growth control and potentially contribute to malignant development. In support of this hypothesis, perturbation of cyclin activity has recently been implicated in the development of several mouse and human tumours (Hunter and Pines 1991) and the ability of E7 to target a cyclin-dependent kinase might also contribute to the oncogenic activity of the virus. It is therefore of particular interest that an E7:kinase association is predominantly seen during G2, suggesting that this might be one of the mechanisms by which E7 advances the cells through these checkpoints in the cell cycle.

5.10   Significance of the E7 interactions with cell proteins

The importance of the interaction between E7 and cell proteins described above has been supported by the study of E7 mutants. The similarity between E7, E1A, and LT is reflected in a region of the three proteins which show strong sequence similarity (Fig. 5.4). Deletion of this region of E7 destroys the ability to form a complex with Rb, p107, or the cdk kinase and more subtle point mutations can also severely inhibit these associations (Davies *et al.* 1993). As expected, E7 proteins unable to bind Rb or p107 fail to alter the E2F-containing complexes (Chellappan *et al.* 1992; Morris *et al.* 1993), but more interestingly all of these mutants are defective in the rodent cell transformation assays (Barbosa *et al.* 1990; Watanabe *et al.* 1990; Phelps *et al.* 1992), indicating that any or all of the viral/cell protein interactions are likely to contribute to the transforming and immortalizing activities of E7. The E7 proteins encoded by the low-risk genital HPV types also show the ability to complex Rb, but with a much reduced efficiency when compared to high-risk E7 proteins. A point mutation converting an amino acid common to the low-risk HPV

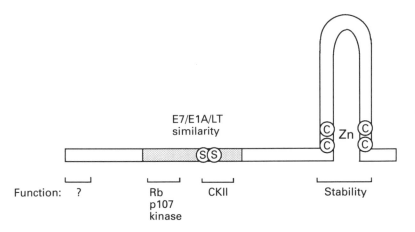

Fig. 5.4 HPV16 E7 protein showing proposed secondary structure involving zinc binding cysteine motif necessary for protein stability. The stippled box shows the position of the sequence similarity between E7, E1A, and LT containing both the Rb, p107, and kinase binding domain and the CKII recognition sequences. The position of the two phosphorylated serine residues within this region is indicated. The unknown activity localized to the N-terminus of the protein is also important for the transforming activity of E7.

E7 proteins to that found at the analogous position in the high-risk HPV types greatly increases the ability of this E7 protein to complex Rb and, significantly, this mutant E7 also acquires the ability to participate in the transformation of rat cells (Heck *et al.* 1992). This strongly supports a role for Rb binding in transformation by E7 and a similar analysis of the ability of the low-risk E7 proteins to associate with p107 or the kinase will certainly be interesting.

Despite the apparent importance of these interactions for E7 function in rodent cells, the significance in human cells is not yet clear. A study of mutant E7 function in human genital epithelial cells indicated that the ability to bind Rb, p107, and the kinase is not necessary for the immortalizing activity of E7 in these cells (Jewers *et al.* 1992). It remains possible that the ability to immortalize human cells is a reflection of an Rb-independent activity of E7, but that subsequent oncogenic conversion depends on this property of the E7 proteins encoded by the high-risk HPV types.

5.11   Additional activities of E7

The concept that other activities of E7 might also be important in human cells is consistent with studies in rodent cells which showed quite clearly that mutants within E7 which do not affect the Rb binding region can still severely reduce transforming activity. The defect in some of these mutants is now understood. Mutations within conserved cysteines found at the carboxy-terminus of E7 (Fig. 5.4) greatly reduce the stability of the protein, making it very difficult to detect in transfected cells (Watanabe *et al.* 1990). These cysteine residues are thought to participate in zinc binding and possibly influence the ability of E7 to form higher-order structures (Roth *et al.* 1992). Recent studies have also indicated that this C-terminal region of E7 is important for disruption of Rb/E2F complexes, although it does not play a role in the binding of E7 to Rb (Huang *et al.* 1993; Wu *et al.* 1993). Two serine residues directly adjacent to the Rb binding sequences (still within the region of similarity to E1A) are targets for phosphorylation by casein kinase II (Fig. 5.4) and mutations of both serines to unphosphorylatable amino acids also severely reduce transforming activity (Barbosa *et al.* 1990; Firzlaff *et al.* 1991). Despite the close proximity to the Rb binding region, phosphorylation and Rb association are independent events and the inability to carry out one of these functions does not impair the other. Interestingly, mutants in which the two serines are substituted by acidic amino acids, which mimic phosphorylated serines, retain transforming activity, suggesting that transformation does not require controlled phosphorylation and dephosphorylation of these sites. Lastly, the extreme N-terminus of E7 is also important for transforming activity since substitutions of the second amino acid almost abolish transforming activity (Fig. 5.4) (Banks *et al.* 1990b; Watanabe *et al.* 1990). The defect in this mutant is unknown; however, the activity which is lost has been shown to be independent of Rb binding both *in vitro* and *in vivo* (Banks *et al.* 1990b; Davies and Vousden 1992). Drawing further analogies with E1A, it is possible that the N-terminus of E7 participates in association with the E1A associated p300 protein, although attempts to demonstrate an association between E7 and p300 have so far been unsuccessful. Identification of the activity affected by this mutant is of particular interest since it potentially provides the key to understanding the mechanism by which E7 contributes to the immortalization of human cells.

5.12   E6 interactions with p53, a monitor of DNA damage

Similarities between the adenoviruses, SV40, and genital HPV types extend to the interaction with another cell protein, p53 (Fig. 5.1). HPV E6, adenovirus E1B, and SV40 LT all form complexes with the p53 protein, although there is no obvious sequence similarity between the three viral proteins and the consequences of the interaction depends on the viral protein involved.

Like Rb, p53 belongs to the class of proteins which negatively control cell growth and can be considered products of tumour suppressor genes. Mutations in the p53 gene are extremely common in many diverse types of human tumours and it is possible that loss of wild type p53 protein is a step in the development of almost all cancers (Hollstein *et al.* 1991). Interestingly, normal cells contain very little p53 protein and it seems that, unlike Rb, p53 does not play a role in progress through a normal cell cycle. Overexpression of p53 results in a block in the cell cycle before entry into DNA synthesis and this growth-arrest function of p53 is implemented in a normal cell in response to DNA damage of the kind induced by UV or gamma irradiation (Kuerbitz *et al.* 1992). The effect of such damage is a sharp rise in p53 levels, achieved by stabilizing the protein, and the consequent arrest in G1 is proposed to allow time for the repair of DNA damage before replication proceeds (Lane 1992). In tumour cells which lack wild type p53, the irradiation-induced G1 arrest does not occur. The damaged DNA is therefore replicated and the consequent acquisition of mutations and gene amplications enhances the risk of malignant conversion. This is almost certainly a simplistic view of the normal function of p53, but the neat way in which this model explains many of the characteristics of p53 makes it likely to be fundamentally correct.

The mechanism by which p53 can induce cell cycle arrest is not clear but appears to be related to the ability of the protein to control transcription of several cellular genes. p53 is a sequence-specific DNA binding protein and the wild type protein can *trans*-activate the expression of genes with p53 binding sites in their regulatory sequences (Funk *et al.* 1992). Less specifically, expression of p53 has been shown to repress transcription from many different cellular promoters (Ginsberg *et al.* 1991). Since the repression does not appear to depend on the specific DNA binding activity of p53, this activity may be indirect and reflect an interaction between p53 and other proteins which participate in the initiation of transcription (Seto *et al.* 1992; Agoff *et al.* 1993). In a cell stressed by DNA damage, therefore, induction of p53 may result in general shutdown of transcription and a resulting cell cycle arrest, with specific activation of genes required to carry out the repair processes.

5.13   Mechanisms of loss of p53 function

There are several ways in which the cell can lose wild type p53 function (Fig. 5.5) (Vogelstein and Kinzler 1992), the most common being point mutation leading to expression of an altered protein. These mutant p53 proteins not only lose suppressor function but can also gain dominant transforming function, which is at least partially explained by a dominant negative activity of the mutant protein which oligomerizes with and thereby

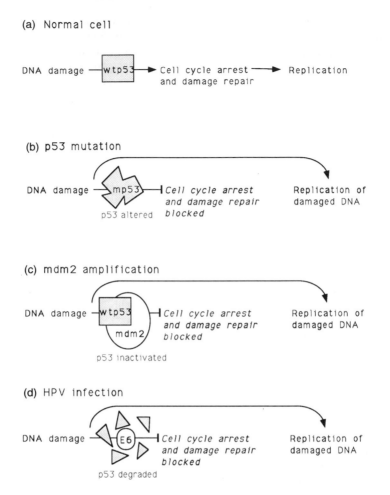

Fig. 5.5 Wild type function of p53 and possible mechanisms by which this can be lost. In a normal cell (a), DNA damage leads to elevation of p53 levels, resulting in cell cycle arrest to allow repair before entry into DNA replication. Loss of this function allows replication of damaged DNA and acquisition of mutations which contribute to oncogenic conversion. Wild type p53 function can be lost by mutation within the p53 gene (b), resulting in expression of a mutant protein, over-expression of mdm2 (c), which complexes with and inactivates wild type p53 or expression of HPV E6 (d), which targets wild type p53 for rapid degradation.

inactivates wild type p53 (Shaulian *et al.* 1992). It is of interest that many of the mutant p53 proteins show loss of both the transcriptional activation and transcriptional repression activities displayed by the wild type protein. However, some of the mutant p53s also acquire an independent transcriptional *trans*-activating activity (Deb *et al.* 1992) which could contribute to the dominant transforming activity displayed by these mutants.

Although mutations within the p53 gene itself are detected in many types of cancers, there are also other, indirect, mechanisms by which p53 function can be lost (Fig. 5.5). One of these involves amplification of the cell gene, *mdm*-2. The mdm2 protein associates with, and inactivates, wild type p53 (Momand *et al.* 1992) and the circumvention of p53 function by mdm2 amplification is frequently seen in sarcomas (Oliner *et al.* 1992). The HPV-associated genital cancers, however, demonstrate a unique mechanism for perturbing wild type p53 function without alterations in cell genes. Infection with a high-risk HPV type and resultant expression of E6 (Fig. 5.5) may have at least some of the same consequences to the cell as mutations within the p53 gene itself, as illustrated by studies showing that E6 can prevent both the transcriptional *trans*-activation and *trans*-repression of wild type p53 (Lechner *et al.* 1992; Mietz *et al.* 1992). The association of p53 with E6 from the high-risk HPV types results in the rapid degradation of p53 (Scheffner *et al.* 1990) and human cells expressing E6 show a marked reduction in the half life of the endogenous p53 (Lechner *et al.* 1992; Hubbert *et al.* 1992). Since the E6 proteins from the low-risk HPV types bind p53 less well and, in *in vitro* assays at least, do not appear to target p53 for degradation, this activity of the high-risk HPV E6 proteins may well be linked to malignant progression. At least one other cell protein, a 100 kD protein, is necessary for the degradation of p53 and this protein can associate with E6 independently of p53 (Huibregtse *et al.* 1991).

The functional significance of the E6:p53 interaction in malignant development is supported by studies of cervical tumour cell lines or primary cervical cancers which show an inverse correlation between the presence of HPV and somatic mutation within the p53 gene (Crook *et al.* 1991; Scheffner *et al.* 1991; Crook *et al.* 1992). These studies indicate that loss of wild type p53 function is important in the development of these malignancies, but that this can be achieved either by alteration of the p53 gene or by infection with a high-risk HPV and expression of E6. Interestingly, there is some evidence that the acquisition of metastatic potential may be accompanied by somatic p53 mutation in an HPV positive, wild type p53 primary tumour (Crook and Vousden 1992). This would be consistent with other studies indicating that at least some mutant p53 proteins display transforming activities which are independent of their ability to inactivate wild type p53.

5.14 Stability of the p53 protein

Although E6 can target p53 for degradation in human cells, expression of E6 in mouse cells has no apparent effect on the half life of the endogenous p53 (Sedman *et al.* 1992) and it is possible that E6 cannot target p53 in murine cells in the same way. This does not appear to be related to an intrinsic inability of E6 to bind to mouse p53 and degradation of the mouse p53 can be demonstrated in *in vitro* assays. It is possible that rodent cells lack a third component, like the 100 kD protein, necessary for efficient degradation. The stability of p53 protein is extremely sensitive to the cell environment and although mutant p53 proteins are generally found to have an increased stability, this may be controlled by surrounding cell factors as much as the structure of the p53 protein itself. In Li-Fraumeni patients who inherit a mutation in one p53 allele, the mutant p53 protein is found stabilized only in tumours that arise following loss of the wild type allele, rather than in the normal somatic cells. Conversely, a cancer family has been described whose normal somatic cells show constitutively high levels of stable wild type p53 proteins (Barnes *et al.* 1992). Similarly, the half life of wild type p53 has been shown to increase in transformed mouse cells. Since one of the important regulations of the activity of p53 itself appears to be at the level of protein stability, the ability of p53 to be targeted for degradation by E6 is particularly interesting. It is not known at present whether E6 enhances the normal mechanism by which p53 is degraded or whether a new pathway is involved. The E6-mediated degradation of p53 utilizes the ubiquitin-dependent proteolytic system which controls the stability of many important growth regulatory proteins within the cell. The ability of fusion proteins containing E6 sequences to target other proteins, apart from p53, for ubiquitin-dependent degradation (Scheffner *et al.* 1992) suggests that the viral protein interfaces directly with this general system of proteolysis. This presents the possibility that E6 also binds and directs the degradation of other, as yet unidentified, cellular proteins.

5.15   Additional activities of E6

Although it does not appear to target p53 for degradation in mouse cells, expression of E6 can participate in the transformation of rodent cells (Sedman *et al.* 1991; Storey and Banks *et al.* 1993), although the activity is weaker than that seen with E7. Some of these studies indicate that p53-independent functions of E6 also contribute to the transforming activity and one of these may be related to the ability of E6 to participate in the control of transcription. E6 has the ability to *trans*-activate both the homologous HPV promoter (Gius *et al.* 1988) as well as several heterologous promoters (Desaintes *et al.* 1992), although it is not known whether these activities are related. It is noteworthy, however, that transformation by bovine papillomavirus type 1 (BPV-1) E6 appears to be dependent on the transcriptional activity of this protein (Lamberti *et al.* 1990). Although less well understood, there is a certain similarity between E6 and E7 in that activities additional to the ability to bind tumour suppressor gene products contribute to transforming activity.

5.16   Other oncoproteins encoded by HPVs

The E6 and E7 genes of the high-risk genital HPV types are obvious candidates for viral oncogenes, since only this portion of the viral genome is consistently conserved and expressed in cancer cells. It is possible, however, that other virally encoded proteins also contribute to the process of onco-genesis, but that their action is required only during a certain stage in malignant development. These genes would therefore act by a mechanism termed 'hit and run', a process which has frequently been postulated to account for the absence of potential viral oncogene products in cancers thought to be associated with viral infection. Examination of the trans-forming proteins encoded by other papillomaviruses shows that the principal oncoprotein encoded by BPV-1, the virus originally used as a model due to its efficient transforming activity, is E5. BPV-1 E5 is an extremely small membrane-associated protein which functions by associating with and stabilizing or activating cell surface receptors such as the PDGF receptor or the EGF receptor (Martin *et al.* 1989; Petti *et al.* 1991). E5-transformed cells become extremely sensitive to exogenous growth factors and the in-creased mitogenic signalling from these activated receptors contributes to uncontrolled growth. Although the HPV E5 proteins are rather dissimilar to BPV-1 E5 at the amino acid level, there is some conservation of overall structure and recent studies indicate HPV16 E5 may function in a similar way (Pim *et al.* 1992).

5.17   Cellular changes contributing to malignant progression

Both experimental and epidemiological studies are in agreement that in-fection with certain HPV types contribute to the development of most cervical cancers and that the action of E6 and E7 participate in malignant progression. The inability of cervical cancer cells to support viral replica-tion, however, illustrates that the oncogenic activities of E6 and E7 do not represent their normal function, which is more likely to be in inducing a cell environment conducive to viral replication. Viewed in this context, the association of E7 with Rb and related proteins might be necessary for the induction of DNA synthesis in an otherwise undividing cervical cell and the ability of E6 to overcome p53 function might remove a checkpoint which would normally detect abnormal DNA replication and induce cell cycle arrest. This rather straightforward model has been refuted recently, however, by studies showing that the Rb binding activity of cottontail papillomavirus is not necessary for wart production (DeFeo-Jones *et al.* 1993). It is possible that loss of control of the expression of E6 and E7, following viral DNA integration, is critical in determining whether the viral proteins contribute to the oncogenic transformation of the infected cell.

Despite the importance of HPV infection there is also evidence that host changes, which might include mutations of oncogenes and tumour suppressor genes within the cervical cell or alterations in the surveillance for abnormalities by the immune system, are necessary to contribute to full malignant progression. Unfortunately, the secondary events contributing to HPV-initiated oncogenesis are not well understood, although some potential candidates have been identified. It is possible that integration of the HPV genome during malignant progression activates cell genes by placing them under the transcriptional control of the virus, and viral integration close to cellular oncogenes has been described (Durst *et al.* 1987). The observation that HPV positive metastases acquire p53 mutations not present in the primary cancers may also reflect an important co-operating event (Crook and Vousden 1992) and it is of interest that mutant p53 can synergize with E7 in the transformation of rodent cells (Crook *et al.* 1991). The contribution of the immune system to cervical cancer development will be discussed in the following chapters.

5.18   HPV oncoproteins as targets for therapeutic intervention

Despite the strong evidence that E6 and E7 contribute to malignant progression, relatively few studies have addressed the important question of whether continued expression of these proteins is necessary for the maintenance of the malignancies. It is possible that infection with HPV simply provides a pool of hyperproliferating cells which are targets for genetic events which participate in malignant transformation. This would be consistent with the apparently early contribution of HPV infection to the malignant process, HPV infection giving rise to pre-malignant lesions which may regress or take decades to progress to an invasive cancer. Such a transient activity of the HPV oncoproteins, however, cannot explain the consistency with which E6 and E7 expression is maintained in cancers and cancer cell lines, suggesting that the expression of these proteins also plays a role in the maintenance of the malignant phenotype. Experimental studies have indicated that loss of E6 and E7 expression in a cancer cell results in the loss of at least some of the transformed characteristics of the cell (von Knebel Doeberitz *et al.* 1988; Steele *et al.* 1992). This is one of the most exciting aspects of HPV research since verification of a continued requirement for E6 and E7 expression would confirm that these viral proteins are perfect targets for anti-cancer drugs or immunotherapies, in addition to their potential in the design of preventative treatments. Since the HPV E6 and E7 proteins have no obvious homologues in mammalian cells, there is real hope that the activity of these viral proteins may be targeted without concomitant deleterious effects on the normal function of cell genes. These approaches are being made possible by our increasing understanding of the molecular basis of the activities displayed by the HPV oncoproteins.

Analysis of the E7 mutants has allowed the design of a 10 amino acid peptide with the same sequence as part of E7, which can prevent the association of E7 with Rb, p107, and the kinase in *in vitro* assays (Jones *et al.* 1990; Davies *et al.* 1993). Since these interactions have been shown to be important for at least some of the oncogenic activities of the E7 protein, such a peptide may form the basis for the design of a drug for the prevention or treatment of HPV-induced cervical tumours. A number of problems remain to be resolved, however, the most pressing at present being to show, in culture, that the peptide can reverse the effects of E7 within a cell. It remains possible that the peptide will mimic, rather than ablate, E7 function and act as an agonist rather than an antagonist of E7. Similarly, the interaction between E6 and p53 could be exploited as a target for the design of therapeutic drugs. Since E5 is not expressed in cancers it is difficult to see how targeting E5 function might be useful for the design of cancer therapies. If this protein does play a role in the early stages of cancer development, however, it may be a good target for intervention to prevent malignant conversion and, since the protein is expressed in the membrane, may be more readily accessible to immunotherapeutic approaches.

The association of certain types of HPV with the development of cervical malignancies is now well established and makes these HPVs the clearest examples of common human tumour viruses. Identification of oncogenes encoded by these viruses has allowed us to begin to understand the molecular mechanisms by which they exert their oncogenic activity and has presented us with exciting targets for the design of prophylactic or therapeutic drugs.

5.19   Summary

The mechanism by which certain types of human papillomaviruses (HPVs) contribute to the development of cervical cancers is related to the expression of the virally encoded E6 and E7 proteins. Both E6 and E7 form complexes with cell proteins which play a role in negatively regulating cell growth. Infection with HPVs and expression of E6 and E7 appears to overcome these blocks to cell proliferation and in some cases may represent one step in the progression to malignancy.

Acknowledgements

I would like to thank Rachel Davies and Fritz Propst for their helpful comments.

References

Agoff, S. N., Hou, J., Linzer, D. I. H., and Wu, B. (1993). Regulation of human hsp70 promoter by p53. *Science*, **259**, 84–7.

Banks, L., Barnett, S. C., and Crook, T. (1990a). HPV-16 E7 functions at the G1 to S phase transition in the cell cycle. *Oncogene*, **5**, 833–37.

Banks, L., Edmonds, C., and Vousden, K. H. (1990b). Ability of the HPV-16 E7 protein to bind RB and induce DNA synthesis is not sufficient for efficient transforming activity. *Oncogene*, **5**, 1383–9.

Barbosa, M. S., Edmonds, C., Fisher, C., Schiller, J. T., Lowy, D. R., and Vousden, K. H. (1990). The region of the HPV E7 oncoprotein homologous to adenovirus E1a and SV40 large T antigen contains separate domains for Rb bindings and casein kinase II phosphorylation. *EMBO Journal*, **9**, 153–60.

Barnes, D. M., Hanby, A. M., Gillett, C. E., Mohammed, S., Hodgson, S., Bobrow, L. G. *et al.* (1992). Abnormal expression of wild type p53 protein in normal cells of a cancer family patient. *Lancet*, **340**, 259–63.

Chellappan, S., Kraus, V., Kroger, B., Münger, K., Howley, P. M., Phelps, W. C. *et al.* (1992). Adenovirus E1A, simian virus 40 tumor antigen, and human papillomavirus E7 protein share the capacity to disrupt the interaction between transcription factor E2F and the retinoblastoma gene product. *Proceedings of the National Academy of Sciences (USA)*, **89**, 4549–53.

Crook, T. and Vousden, K. H. (1992). Properties of p53 mutations detected in primary and secondary cervical cancers suggests mechanisms of metastasis and involvement of environmental carcinogens. *European Molecular Biology Organisation Journal*, **11**, 3935–40.

Crook, T., Fisher, C., and Vousden, K. H. (1991a). Modulation of immortalizing properties of human papillomavirus type 16 E7 by p53 expression. *Journal of Virology*, **65**, 505–10.

Crook, T., Wrede, D., and Vousden, K. H. (1991b). p53 point mutation in human papillomavirus negative cervical carcinoma cell lines. *Oncogene*, **6**, 873–5.

Crook, T., Wrede, D., Tidy, J. A., Mason, W. P., Evans, D. J., and Vousden, K. H. (1992). Clonal p53 mutation in primary cervical cancer: association with human-papillomavirus-negative tumours. *Lancet*, **339**, 1070–3.

Dalton, S. (1992). Cell cycle regulation of the human *cdc2* gene. *European Molecular Biology Organisation Journal*, **11**, 1797–804.

Davies, R. C. and Vousden, K. H. (1992). Functional analysis of human papillomavirus type 16 E7 by complementation with adenovirus E1a mutants. *Journal of General Virology*, **73**, 2135–9.

Davies, R., Hicks, R., Crook, T., Morris, J., and Vousden, K. H. (1993). Association of E7 with a histone H1 kinase activity and p107 correlates with transformation. *Journal of Virology*, **67**, 2521–8.

Deb, S., Jackson, C. T., Subler, M. A., and Martin, D. W. (1992). Modulation of cellular and viral promoters by mutant human p53 proteins found in tumor cells. *Journal of Virology*, **66**, 6164–70.

DeFeo-Jones, D., Vuoculo, G. A., Haskall, K. M., Hannobik, M. G., Kiefer. D. M. *et al.* (1993). Papillomavirus E7 protein binding to the retinoblastoma protein is not required for viral induction of warts. *Journal of Virology*, **67**, 716–25.

Desaintes, C., Hallez, S., van Alphen, P., and Burny, A. (1992). Transcriptional activation of several heterologous promoters by the E6 protein of human papillomavirus type 16. *Journal of Virology*, **66**, 325–33.

Dyson, N., Guida, P., Münger, K., and Harlow, E. (1992). Homologous sequences in adenovirus E1A and human papillomavirus E7 proteins mediate interaction with the same set of cellular proteins. *Journal of Virology*, **66**, 6893–902.

Durst, M., Croce, C. M., Gissmann, L., Schwarz, E., and Huebner, K. (1987). Papillomavirus sequences integrate near cellular oncogenes in some cervical carcinomas. *Proceedings of the National Academy of Sciences (USA)*, **84**, 1070–4.

Firzlaff, J. M., Luscher, B., and Eisenman, R. N. (1991). Negative charge at the casein kinase II phosphorylation site is important for transformation but not for Rb protein binding by the E7 protein of human papillomavirus type 16. *Proceedings of the National Academy of Sciences (USA)*, **88**, 5187–91.

Funk, W. D., Pak, D. T., Karas, R. H., Wright, W. E., and Shay, J. W. (1992). A transcriptionally active DNA-binding site for human p53 protein complexes. *Molecular Cell Biology*, **12**, 2866–71.

Ginsberg, D., Mechta, F., Yaniv, M., and Oren, M. (1991). Wild-type p53 can down-modulate the activity of various promoters. *Proceedings of the National Academy of Sciences (USA)*, **88**, 9979–83.

Gius, G., Grossman, S., Bedell, M. A., and Laimins, L. A. (1988). Inducible and constitutive enhancer domains in the noncoding region of human papillomavirus type 18. *Journal of Virology*, **62**, 665–72.

Goodrich, D. W., Wang, N. P., Qian, Y.-W., Lee, Y.-H. P., and Lee, W.-H. (1991). The retinoblastoma gene product regulates progression through the G1 phase of the cell cycle. *Cell*, **67**, 293–302.

Green, M. R. (1989). When the products of oncogenes and anti-oncogenes meet. *Cell*, **56**, 1–3.

Gu, W., Schneider, J. W., Condorelli, G., Kaushal, S., Mahdavi, V. and Nadal-Ginard, B. (1993). Interaction of myogenic factors and retinoblastoma protein mediates muscle cell commitment and differentiation. *Cell*, **72**, 309–24.

Halbert, C. L., Demers, G. W., and Galloway, D. A. (1992). The E6 and E7 genes of human papillomavirus type 6 have weak immortalizing activity in human epithelial cells. *Journal of Virology*, **66**, 2125–34.

Hamel, P. A., Gallie, B. L., and Phillips, R. A. (1992a). The retinoblastoma protein and cell cycle regulation. *Trends in Genetics*, **8**, 180–5.

Hamel, P. A., Gill, R. M., Phillips, R. A., and Gallie, B. A. (1992b). Transcriptional repression of the E2-containing promoters EIIaE, c-*myc*, and RB1 by the product of the *RB* gene. *Molecular Cell Biology*, **12**, 3431–8.

Hawley-Nelson, P., Vousden, K. H., Hubbert, N. L., Lowy, D. R., and Schiller, J. T. (1989). HPV16 E6 and E7 proteins cooperate to immortalize human foreskin keratinocytes. *European Molecular Biology Organisation Journal*, **8**, 3905–10.

Heck, D. V., Yee, C. L., Howley, P. M., and Münger, K. (1992). Efficiency of binding the retinoblastoma protein correlates with the transforming capacity of the E7 oncoproteins of the human papillomaviruses. *Proceedings of the National Academy of Sciences (USA)*, **89**, 4442–6.

Hollstein, M., Sidransky, D., Vogelstein, B., and Harris, C. C. (1991). p53 mutations in human cancers. *Science*, **253**, 49–53.

Hubbert, N. L., Sedman, S. A., and Schiller, J. T. (1992). Human papillomavirus type 16 E6 increases the degradation rate of p53 in human keratinocytes. *Journal of Virology*, **66**, 6237–41.

Hudson, J. B., Bedell, M. A., McCance, D. J., and Laimins, L. A. (1990). Immortalisation and altered differentiation of human keratinocytes *in vitro* by the E6 and E7 open reading frames of human papillomavirus type 18. *Journal of Virology*, **64**, 519–26.

Huang, P. S., Patrick, D. R., Edwards, G., Goodhart, P. J., Huber, H. E., Miles, L. *et al.* (1993). Protein domains governing interactions between E2F, the retinoblastoma gene product, and the human papillomavirus type 16 E7 protein. *Molecular Cell Biology*, **139**, 953–60.

Huibregtse, J. M., Scheffner, M., and Howley, P. M. (1991). A cellular protein mediates association of p53 with the E6 oncoprotein of human papillomavirus types 16 or 18. *European Molecular Biology Organisation Journal*, **10**, 4129–35.

Hunter, T. and Pines, J. (1991). Cyclins and cancer. *Cell*, **66**, 1071–4.

Jewers, R. J., Hildebrandt, P., Ludlow, J. W., Kell, B., and McCance, D. J. (1992). Regions of HPV 16 E7 oncoprotein required for immortalization of human keratinocytes. *Journal of Virology*, **66**, 1329–35.

Jones, R. E., Wegrzyn, R. J., Patrick, D. R., Balishin, N. L., Vuocolo, G. A., Riemen, M. W. *et al.* (1990). Identification of HPV-16 E7 peptides that are potent antagonists of E7 binding to the retinoblastoma suppressor protein. *Journal of Biological Chemistry*, **265**, 12782–5.

Kim, S.-J., Onwuta, U. S., Lee, Y. I., Li, R., Botchan, M. R., and Robbins, P. D. (1992). The retinoblastoma gene product regulates Sp-1-mediated transcription. *Molecular Cell Biology*, **12**, 2455–63.

Knudson, A. G. Jr. (1971). Mutation and cancer: statistical study of retinoblastoma. *Proceedings of the National Academy of Sciences (USA)*, **68**, 820–3.

Kuerbitz, S. J., Plunkett, B. S., Walsh, W. V., and Kastan, M. B. (1992). Wild-type p53 is a cell cycle checkpoint determinant following irradiation. *Proceedings of the National Academy of Sciences (USA)*, **89**, 7491–5.

Lamberti, C., Morrissey, L. C., Grossman, S. R., and Androphy, E. J. (1990). Transcriptional activation by the papillomavirus E6 zinc finger oncoprotein. *European Molecular Biology Organisation Journal*, **9**, 1907–13.

Lane, D. P. (1992). p53, guardian of the genome. *Nature*, **358**, 15–16.

Lechner, M. S., Mack, D. H., Finicle, A. B., Crook, T., Vousden, K. H., and Laimins, L. A. (1992). Human papillomavirus E6 proteins bind p53 *in vivo* and abrogate p53 mediated repression of transcription. *European Molecular Biology Organisation Journal*, **11**, 3045–52.

Marshall, C. J. (1991). Tumor suppressor genes. *Cell*, **64**, 313–26.

Martin, P., Vass, W. C., Schiller, J. T., Lowy, D. R., and Velu, T. J. (1989). The bovine papillomavirus E5 transforming protein can stimulate the transforming activity of EGF and CSF-1 receptors. *Cell*, **59**, 21–32.

McKinney, J. D. and Heintz, N. (1991). Transcriptional regulation in the eukaryotic cell cycle. *Trends in Biochemical Sciences*, **16**, 430–1.

Mietz, J. A., Unger, T., Huibregtse, J. M., and Howley, P. M. (1992). The transcriptional transactivation function of wild type p53 is inhibited by SV40 large T-antigen and by HPV-16 E6 oncoprotein. European *Molecular Biology Organisation Journal*, **11**, 5013–20.

Momand, J., Zambetti, G. P., Olson, D. C., George, D., and Levine, A. J. (1992). The *mdm*-2 oncogene product forms a complex with the p53 protein and inhibits p53-mediated transactivation. *Cell*, **69**, 1237–45.

Morris, J. D. H., Crook, T., Bandara, L. R., Davies, R. La Thangue, N. B. and Vousden, K. H. (1993). Human papillomavirus 16 E7 regulates E2F and contributes to mitogenic signalling. *Oncogene*, **8**, 893–8.

Murray, A. W. (1992). Creative blocks: cell-cycle checkpoints and feedback controls. *Nature*, **359**, 599–604.

Münger, K., Phelps, W. C., Bubb, V., Howley, P. M., and Schlegel, R. (1989). The E6 and E7 genes of the human papillomavirus type 16 together are necessary and sufficient for transformation of primary human keratinocytes. *Journal of Virology*, **63**, 4417–21.

Oliner, J. D., Kinzler, K. W., Meltzer, P. S., George, D. L., and Vogelstein, B. (1992). Amplification of a gene encoding a p53-associated protein in human sarcomas. *Nature*, **358**, 80–3.

Petti, L., Nilson, L. A., and Dimaio, D. (1991). Activation of the platelet-derived growth factor receptor by the bovine papillomavirus E5 transforming protein. *European Molecular Biology Organisation Journal*, **10**, 845–55.

Phelps, W. C., Bagchi, S., Barnes, J. A., Raychaudhuri, P., Kraus, V., Münger, K. *et al.* (1991). Analysis of *trans* activation by human papillomavirus type 16 E7 and adenovirus 12S E1A suggests a common mechanism. *Journal of Virology*, **65**, 6922–30.

Phelps, W. C., Münger, K., Yee, C. L., Barnes, J. A., and Howley, P. M. (1992). Structure-function analysis of the human papillomavirus type 16 E7 oncoprotein. *Journal of Virology*, **66**, 2418–27.

Pim, D., Collins, M., and Banks, L. (1992). Human papillomavirus type 16 E5 gene stimulates the transforming activity of the epidermal growth factor receptor. *Oncogene*, **7**, 27–32.

Pines, J. and Hunter, T. (1991). Cyclin-dependent kinases: a new cell cycle motif? *Trends in Cell Biology*, **1**, 117–212.

Roth, E. J., Kurz, B., Liang, L., Hansen, C. L., Dameron, C. T., Winge, D. R. *et al.* (1992). Metal thiolate coordination in the E7 proteins of human papilloma virus 16 and cottontail rabbit papilloma virus as expressed in Escherichia coli. *Journal of Biological Chemistry*, **267**, 16390–5.

Sato, H., Furuno, A., and Yoshiike, K. (1989). Expression of human papillomavirus type 16 E7 gene induces DNA synthesis of rat 3Y1 cells. *Virology*, **168**, 195–9.

Scheffner, M., Werness, B. A., Huibregtse, J. M., Levine, A. J., and Howley, P. M. (1990). The E6 oncoprotein encoded by human papillomavirus types 16 and 18 promotes the degradation of p53. *Cell*, **63**, 1129–36.

Scheffner, M., Münger, K., Byrne, J. C., and Howley, P. M. (1991). The state of the p53 and retinoblastoma genes in human cervical carcinoma cell lines. *Proceedings of the National Academy of Sciences (USA)*, **88**, 5523–7.

Scheffner, M., Münger, K., Huibregtse, J. M., and Howley, P. M. (1992). Targeted degradation of the retinoblastoma protein by human papillomavirus E7-E6 fusion proteins. *European Molecular Biology Organisation Journal*, **11**, 2425–31.

Schwartz, J. K., Devoto, S. H., Smith, E. J., Chellapan, S. P., Jakoi, L. and Nevins, J. R. (1993). Interactions of the p107 and Rb protein with E2F during the cell proliferation response. *European Molecular Biology Organisation Journal*, **12**, 1013–20.

Sedman, S. A., Barbosa, M. S., Vass, W. C., Hubbert, N. L., Haas, J. A., Lowy, D. R. *et al.* (1991). The full-length E6 protein of human papillomavirus type 16 has transforming and *trans*-activating activities and cooperates with E7 to immortalize keratinocytes in culture. *Journal of Virology*, **65**, 4860–6.

Sedman, S., Hubbert, N. L., Vass, W. C., Lowy, D. R., and Schiller, J. T. (1992). Mutant p53 can substitute for human papillomavirus type 16 E6 in immortalization of human keratinocytes but does not have E6-associated *trans*-activation or transforming activity. *Journal of Virology*, **66**, 4201–8.

Seto, E., Usheva, A., Zambetti, G. P., Momand, J., Horikoshi, N., Weinmann, R. *et al.* (1992). Wild-type p53 binds to the TATA-binding protein and represses transcription. *Proceedings of the National Academy of Sciences (USA)*, **89**, 12028–32.

Shaulian, E., Zauberman, A., Ginsberg, D., and Oren, M. (1992). Identification of a minimal transforming domain of p53: negative dominance through abrogation of sequence specific DNA binding. *Molecular Cell Biology*, **12**, 5581–92.

Steele, C., Sacks, P. G., Alder-Stortkz, K., and Shillitoe, E. J. (1992). Effect on cancer cells of plasmids that express antisense RNA of human papilloma virus type 18. *Cancer Research*, **52**, 4706–11.

Storey, A. and Banks, L. (1993). Human papillomavirus type 16 E6 gene cooperates with EJ-*ras* to immortalize primary mouse cells. *Oncogene*, **8**, 919–24.

Tommasino, M., Adamczewski, J. P., Carlotti, F., Barth, C. F., Contorni, M., Cavalieri, F. *et al.* (1993). HPV16 E7 protein associates with the protein kinase p33^{CDK2} and cyclin A. *Oncogene*, **8**, 195–202.

Vogelstein, B. and Kinzler, K. W. (1992). p53 function and dysfunction. *Cell*, **70**, 523–6.

von Knebel Doeberitz, M., Oltersdorf, T., Schwarz, E., and Gissmann, L. (1988). Correlation of modified human papilloma virus early gene expression with altered growth properties in C4-1 cervical carcinoma cells. *Cancer Research*, **48**, 3780–6.

Vousden, K. H. (1991a). Papillomaviruses and assays for transforming genes. In *Methods in molecular biology* (ed. M. Collins), Vol.8, pp. 159–74. Humana Press, Clifton, NJ.

Vousden, K. H. (1991b). Human papillomavirus transforming genes. *Seminars in Virology*, **2**, 307–17.

Vousden, K. H. and Jat, P. M. (1989). Functional similarity between HPV16 E7, SV40 large T and adenovirus E1a proteins. *Oncogene*, **4**, 153–8.

Watanabe, S., Kanda, T., Sato, H., Furuno, A., and Yoshiike, K. (1990). Mutational analysis of human papillomavirus type 16 E7 functions. *Journal of Virology*, **64**, 207–14.

Wientraub, S. J., Prater, C. A., and Dean, D. C. (1992). Retinoblastoma protein switches the E2F site from positive to negative element. *Nature*, **358**, 259–61.

Wu, E. W., Clemens, K. E., Heck, D. V., and Münger, K. (1993). The human papillomavirus E7 oncoprotein and cellular transcription factor E2F bind to separate sites on the retinoblastoma tumour suppressor protein. *Journal of Virology*, **67**, 2402–7.

Xiong, Y. and Beach, D. (1991). Population explosion in the cyclin family. *Current Biology*, **1**, 362–4.

6 Virus-keratinocyte interactions in the infectious cycle

MARGARET A. STANLEY

6.1 Introduction

There seems to be little doubt that infection with certain types of HPV, the so-called 'oncogenic HPVs' 16, 18, 31, 33, and 35, is the major but not the only risk factor in the subsequent development of cervical cancer (Schiffmann 1992). This has raised the possibility that if one could prevent infection with HPV or treat established HPV infections this would prevent the development of HPV-associated cancer and be an effective anti-cancer strategy. Other chapters in this book address the feasibility of this exercise from the immunological perspective but any understanding of the immune responses to the genital HPVs and the implementation of prophylactic or therapeutic strategies is absolutely dependent upon a knowledge of the biology of the virus and its interaction with the target cell for infection, the keratinocyte. Despite some important advances in the past 2–3 years this information remains fragmentary because of the unique replication strategy of HPV—a strategy in which virus replication and differentiation proceed in parallel and in which vegetative viral growth occurs only in a terminally differentiating epithelium. The difficulties of reproducing this scenario *in vitro* have contributed significantly to the problems in understanding papillomavirus—keratinocyte interactions and the regulation of viral gene expression during permissive growth.

6.2 Keratinocyte lineage and the regulation of terminal differentiation

Since the life history of the keratinocyte and the infectious cycle of HPVs are interdependent, before discussing what is known of the latter it is worth briefly considering the kinetic organization of squamous epithelium and the regulation of keratinocyte differentiation. Stratified squamous epithelium is basically of two types: non-keratinizing covering the internal wet mucosae such as the female genital tract, and the keratinizing epithelium of the skin. All squamous epithelium has the same basic structure and can be divided into several zones:

(1) the basal layer or stratum basale, small cylindrical cells with large nuclei;

(2) the prickle cell or stratum spinosum, several layers of polyhedral cells with prominent intercellular junctions;

(3) the granular layer or stratum granulosum packed polyhedral cells rich in keratohyalin granules;

(4) the stratum corneum, a superficial layer of elongated flattened enucleate squames.

In non-keratinizing epithelia the stratum corneum is not present, cells flatten as they migrate and the nucleus becomes smaller and pycnotic. Keratinocytes, characterized by an intermediate filament network of keratin polypeptides, comprise more than 95 per cent of the resident squamous epithelial population, the remaining 5 per cent being made up of melanocytes, Merkel cells, and Langerhans cells, the antigen-presenting cells of the epithelium. In addition there are peripatetic intra-epithelial populations of immunocytes including $CD4^+$ and $CD8^+$ lymphocytes and macrophages.

The keratinocytes constitute a self-renewing population with the basal keratinocytes forming the proliferative compartment; cells migrate from this layer, differentiating as they progress upwards to be exfoliated or desquamated from the surface and replaced by new cells from below. Such a self-renewing population by definition contains a subset of cells with stem cell properties and there is therefore a keratinocyte lineage which ranges from the primitive stem cell in the basal layer through to the terminally differentiated enucleate squame. The lineage has a structural organization seen at its most marked in slowly renewing epidermal populations. Here the cells are arranged in hexagonally shaped columns or stacks known as epidermal proliferative units or EPU. Each EPU has a basal layer of about 10 keratinocytes, at the centre of which is a Langerhans cell (Potten 1974). The most central keratinocyte in this layer has the properties of a putative stem cell—it is a slow-cycling, label-retaining cell (Morris *et al.* 1985). The peripheral basal cells in the EPU are mitotically active but with a limited proliferative capacity and represent the mature progeny of the stem cell which have migrated from the centre of the EPU to the periphery. These peripheral cells will then migrate upward, entering the differentiation programme.

The evolution of the basal keratinocyte to a terminally differentiated cornified cell is associated with the sequential induction of a family of differentiation specific proteins, both structural and regulatory, which are specific to keratinocytes. Morphological changes are a striking feature of the differentiating epithelium and these reflect changes in the keratin poly-peptides which comprise the intermediate filament network. Basal epidermal keratinocytes have an IF network consisting of a 1:1 ratio of keratins 5 and 14 (Nelson and Sun 1983); in cervical keratinocytes K19 is also expressed (Dixon and Stanley 1984). Movement into the spinous layers is accompanied by the expression of new keratins K1 and K10 in the epidermis and K13 and K4 in the ectocervix (Moll *et al.* 1982). Not only are new keratins synthesized in the spinous layers but the physical arrangement of the polymer changes and they aggregate into thin bundles, the tonofilaments. A characteristic of differentiated keratinocytes is the cornified envelope, a 12 nm thick band apposed to the cytoplasmic side of the plasma membrane; this envelope results from the cross-linking of glutamine-rich, lysine-rich proteins such as involucrin, a 92kd species (Rice and Green 1979). Involucrin synthesis is a specific marker of keratinocyte differentiation since the protein is not synthesized in any significant amounts in any other cell types. In non-keratinizing epithelia, the spinous and granular layers are characterized by the accumulation of intra-cytoplasmic glycogen, the distribution of which in the cervix parallels that of involucrin. The rigidity of squamous epithelium is of functional importance and contributing to this are the desmosomes, members of the calcium-dependent cadherin family of intercellular adhesion molecules, which interconnect cells of the basal and spinous zones into a tight three-dimensional lattice. The desmosomal proteins show a differentiation dependence with basal-specific and differentiation-specific species. When the spinous cells reach the granular layer the protein synthetic profile changes; there is a decrease in keratin and involucrin synthesis and the production of a new protein, filaggrin, which binds to the keratin tonofilaments forming thick macrofibrillar cables (Rothnagel and Steinert 1990). Another late differentiation protein is loricrin, a component of the rigid cornified envelope of the terminally differentiated keratinocyte and cross-linked into the envelope by the activation of the keratinocyte-specific transglutaminase (reviewed in Polakwska and Goldsmith 1991).

At the mRNA level expression of keratinocyte markers is rigidly compartmentalized, with the induction of certain genes tightly coupled to the repression of others. A good example of this is the regulation of expression of the keratins. K5 and K14 mRNAs are abundant in basal cells but markedly reduced in spinous cells when K1 and K10 are induced (Stoler *et al.* 1988); K1 and K10 mRNAs are decreased when loricrin and filaggrin are induced (Mehrel *et al.* 1990). There is no doubt that extracellular calcium levels are a major regulator of these processes and recent studies have provided strong evidence that the central player in the spinous to granular transition both at the transcriptional and translational level is protein kinase C activated by Ca^{++} (Duglosz and Yuspa 1993). The journey from the basal layer to the surface is not achieved overnight and certainly in skin the most conservative estimate is that 14 days is the minimum turnover time for epithelial renewal. Non-keratinizing epithelia such as the cervix may have a more rapid turnover time but this is unlikely to be less than 7–10 days.

6.3   The infectious cycle of HPV

The papillomaviruses exhibit an exquisite tissue tropism. They are strictly epitheliotropic viruses and they have evolved a unique replication strategy which depends absolutely upon the differentiation programme of the target cell for infection—the keratinocyte. Only keratinocytes (or cells with the potential for keratinocyte maturation) can be infected and only in the terminally differentiating keratinocyte are viral capsid proteins synthesized and viral particles assembled. This absolute dependence upon the micro-environment provided by differentiating epithelium for infection, replication, and assembly was first demonstrated for an animal papillomavirus, the cotton tail rabbit virus, CRPV (Kreider and Bartlett 1981). The basal or germinal layers of the rabbit papillomas contain proliferating cells but viral DNA cannot be detected in these cells. In the upper layers of the stratum spinosum and in the granulosum virus DNA at high copy number can be detected but viral capsid antigen and viral particles can be detected only in the extreme superficial differentiated layers of the papilloma. This pattern of replication and dependence upon epithelial differentiation for late gene expression has been shown also for HPV in HPV 6 and 11 induced condyloma (Stoler *et al.* 1986, 1989) and for low-grade cervical intra-epithelial lesions (Higgins *et al.* 1992, Stoler *et al.* 1992).

These studies, however, do not give information on the temporal aspects of viral gene expression, information which for most viruses comes from *in vitro* studies on the infectious cycle, but to date no *in vitro* system has been described which supports the complete infectious cycle of an HPV. However, viral gene expression during the infectious cycle of HPV 11 has been analysed using the nude mouse xenograft model developed by Kreider and his colleagues (Kreider *et al.* 1985). In this system small chips of foreskin or cervical epithelium are incubated with the Hershey strain of HPV 11 for 1–2 hours *in vitro*. The chips are then implanted under the renal capsule of the nude mouse where after some time condylomatous transformation of the grafts occurs with the production of large amounts of virions (Kreider *et al.* 1985, 1986). The Hershey strain has been serially passaged using this technique and the organotropism of HPV 11 examined by infecting skin from different body sites; foreskin and urethral skin supporting viral growth most effectively.

Viral gene expression during the infectious cycle in this system has been examined by RNA:RNA *in situ* hybridization using exon-specific probes and immunohistochemistry (Stoler 1990). In the first four weeks after infection and grafting of skin chips no viral activity is detectable. Viral DNA cannot be detected, which suggests that viral copy number in the infected cells is below 50 copies/cell. The first detectable signals in the experimental condyloma were seen at four weeks with expression from probes which spanned the early region in general and the E4/E5 region in particular. In the 4–8 week period post grafting there were dramatic changes in morphology, viral DNA replication, and mRNA transcription. The implants underwent condylomatous transformation with the characteristic increase in the proliferative compartment of the epithelium and koilocytosis and parakeratosis of the superficial layers. Viral DNA replication increased with cellular differentiation and was detectable first in the stratum spinosum but with a maximal signal in the stratum granulosum. E6/E7 transcripts were not detected in basal cells but appeared in the parabasal layers at week six, becoming progressively more abundant with time. Transcripts for the capsid proteins L1 and L2 did not appear until week eight and were confined to the most superficial differentiated cells and immunocytochemistry using antisera to the group-specific antigen revealed that L1 mRNA expressing cells were antigen positive.

This dependence upon the differentiated environment for late gene expression has also been shown for HPV 16 using the W12 keratinocyte cell line (Stanley *et al.* 1989). These cells were derived from a low-grade cervical lesion and are an established but non-malignant keratinocyte cell line containing on average 100 copies/cell of HPV 16 predominantly in episomal form. In submerged culture these cells undergo limited stratification, express basal keratins (19,5,14,16,17), but do not express any markers of terminal differentiation. HPV early region genes are transcribed and E6 and E7 proteins synthesized at low levels. Late gene transcripts are present in trace amounts and this is attributable to the presence of rare cells with very high viral copy number (Higgins and Stanley, unpublished data). Transplantation of W12 cells to a skin pocket on the flank of the nude mouse using a transplantation technique which permits epithelial reformation results in the expression of the differentiated phenotype by W12 cells and major changes in HPV 16 gene expression. These changes, as in the HPV 11 induced experimental condyloma, are time dependent. Ten days after grafting W12 cells have reformed an epithelium which morphologically appears identical to normal ectocervical epithelium; at this time viral sequences cannot be detected by DNA:DNA *in situ* hybridization. At four weeks post grafting the epithelium has thickened and has the histological appearance of a CIN1/2 lesion. Viral DNA sequences can be identified in the superficial cells and immunohistochemistry reveals isolated cells positive for the L1 capsid antigen. At six weeks post grafting many cells are positive for the L1 capsid antigen, the E4 protein is expressed throughout the stratum granulosum and viral particles can be identified in the degenerating nuclei close to the keratinized superficial layers of the grafts (Sterling *et al.* 1990), and immunostaining with anti-E4 and L1 antibodies and transmission electron microscopy confirm that these viral particles are HPV 16 (Sterling *et al.* 1993). The histological appearance of the four and six week W12 grafts are comparable to the histological appearance of clinical CIN lesions but differ in that they exhibit extensive hyperkeratosis. Clinical cervical lesions rarely contain viral particles to any significant level, they do not exhibit hyperkeratosis, and it seems probable that productively infected squames are exfoliated in the natural infection releasing infectious particles into the cervical and vaginal secretions.

6.4 *In vitro* culture of HPV

In vitro systems which permit serial passage of keratinocytes were first described by Rheinwald and Green (1975) in a seminal series of experiments. Infection of such monolayer cultures of keratinocytes with HPV virions or transfection with HPV DNA has been disappointing, with transient replication only of the episomes and rapid loss of DNA from the cells (Mungal *et al.* 1992). Transfection of cloned DNA from the oncogenic HPVs together with a selectable marker has consistently resulted in the derivation of immortal lines in which viral DNA is integrated, making such cells useless for studies on episomal replication. Two cell lines the W12 line (Stanley *et al.* 1989) and CIN 612 (Bedell *et al.* 1991) in which the viral DNA is present as the episome have been derived as a rare event when low-grade clinical biopsies have been cultured *in vitro*.

The infectious cycle of the papillomaviruses is absolutely dependent upon the regulated lineage expression of the keratinocyte 'from the cradle to the grave', so to speak, and *in vitro* systems permissive for HPV must mimic the environment which supports the complete keratinocyte differentiation programme. The regulation of keratinocyte differentiation is extremely complex but depends very significantly on signals from the extracellular matrix of the sub-epithelial stroma or dermis. Culture systems which partially reproduce this connective tissue matrix have been developed. In essence all these systems consist of a collagen matrix seeded with fibroblasts of murine or human origin. Keratinocytes are seeded thickly onto this matrix in submerged culture and when confluent the collagen keratinocyte matrix is raised by placing on an inert support (usually a stainless steel grid) so that the keratinocyte layer is at the air–liquid interface. In such organotypic or 'raft' cultures the keratinocytes stratify and differentiate with the expression of the differentiation-specific keratins (Merrick *et al.* 1992).

In such organotypic cultures, immortal keratinocyte cell lines derived by transfection or electroporation with cloned HPV 16 or 18 DNA can be shown to stratify and undergo abnormal differentiation comparable to those seen in CIN *in vivo*. Cell lines containing episomal copies of HPV, the W12 and CIN 612 lines, stratify and differentiate and viral DNA amplification can be shown, by in situ hybridization, to occur in the upper layers of the stratified cells (Bedell *et al.* 1991). Transcriptional analysis of HPV 31b in the CIN 612 line in organotypic culture shows significant differences compared to monolayer cultures with evidence for a novel promoter, p742 in the E7 gene from which abundant E1^E4 and E5 transcripts are initiated (Hummel *et al.* 1992). Recent developments with organotypic cultures have achieved permissive HPV replication and viral assembly *in vitro* when keratinocytes containing HPV as the episome are used to initiate the cultures. Dollard and colleagues (1992) explanted small fragments of HPV 11 containing condylomas (generated as nude mouse xenografts) onto collagen matrices seeded with A31 3T3 fibroblasts. Keratinocytes grew out from these explanted fragments, stratified and differentiated and within three weeks of culture complete viral transcription and replication leading to viral assembly occurred. Viral gene expression in this system is exquisitely dependent upon the source of the fibroblasts in the collagen matrix. Thus if the matrices are seeded with human dermal fibroblasts no viral DNA amplification, late gene expression, or virion assembly can be demonstrated and seeding with the A31 3T3 strain of mouse fibroblasts is essential for permissive viral growth. Viral gene expression in these permissive organotypic cultures was virtually identical to that seen in the clinical biopsies and in the experimental condyloma in the nude mouse with high copy viral DNA and abundant E6/E7 mRNAs in the upper spinous layers.

The abundant expression of E6/E7 message in non-proliferating differentiated cells is of considerable interest, suggesting that these viral gene products play an important role in vegetative viral DNA replication, probably by inducing the expression of cellular genes required for viral DNA synthesis. One such cellular gene appears to be proliferating cell nuclear antigen PCNA, an accessory protein for DNA polymerase δ. In the raft cultures permissive for HPV-11 viral replication, PCNA antigen was induced in the differentiating layers in parallel with viral DNA amplification. This expression of PCNA in the experimental system reproduces observations *in vivo* in low-grade CIN and condyloma acuminata which show a consistent expression of PCNA in the upper spinous layer (Demeter *et al.*, in press). Support for the suggestion that viral gene products induce PCNA expression has come from experiments in which recombinant retroviruses containing the entire URR of HPV 18 and various combinations of the E6 and E7 ORFS were used to infect primary human keratinocytes. When the cells infected with constructs which permitted expression of the wild type E7 protein were grown in organotypic culture, PCNA induction in the differentiated spinous layer keratinocytes was observed (Cheng *et al.*, personal communication).

A different approach for the induction of the completely differentiated phenotype in raft culture has been taken by Meyer and colleagues (1992). In these studies the CIN 612 cell line which contains episomal copies of HPV 31b were grown in organotypic cultures pulsed with the phorbol ester TPA (Tetradecanoylphorbol-13-Acetate), a potent activator of PKC. Such treatment resulted in an abrupt spinous to granular transition in the upper layers of the cultures, the induction of capsid protein synthesis and the production of HPV 31b virions which could be purified by density gradient separation. Similarly TPA treatment of organotypic cultures of the W12 line results in a massive induction of L1 and L2 messages in these cells and the synthesis of capsid proteins (Higgins and Stanley, unpublished data).

The effects of TPA in this system in which the specific activation of PKC induces the abrupt spinous to granular transition and permits capsid protein synthesis are of considerable interest. The available evidence strongly suggests that PKC selectively triggers the late stage of keratinocyte differentiation at which early marker expression is repressed and late markers induced (Dlugosz and Yuspa 1993). The expression of certain keratins is regulated at the post-transcriptional level and transcriptional destabilization may be required for the rapid disappearance of, for example, the K1 transcripts in cells entering the granular compartment (Stoler *et al.* 1988). In contrast loricrin and filaggrin expression is induced at this time but whether the regulation of this is at the transcriptional or post-transcriptional level is not clear at the moment. TPA influences mRNA stability in several systems, either increasing (Weber *et al.* 1989) or decreasing transcript half-life (Zhu *et al.* 1991) and a protein factor appears to be involved in some of these instances. There is evidence that the regulation of expression of HPV 16 L1 is at the level of RNA processing. A negative regulatory element has been identified in the HPV 16 late region around position 7128 close to the L1 stop codon (Kennedy *et al.* 1991). This negative element can act to destabilize poly A^+ RNA; it is functional in basal cells and cross-links with a 64kd cellular protein (Kennedy, personal communication) and one might speculate that L1 transcript stabilization requires the inactivation of this negative element and that this is one of the consequences of PKC activation.

6.5 The target cell for infection

The recent developments in *in vitro* culture of HPVs are extremely encouraging but the fact remains that at present virions generated *in vitro* have not been shown to be capable of infecting keratinocytes and inducing another round of replication *in vitro*. This inability to infect with virus and initiate episomal replication *in vitro* parallels many unsuccessful attempts to introduce cloned viral DNA into keratinocytes and elicit viral replication and this raizes the issue of the nature of the target cell for infection. It is clear that basal keratinocytes are infected but are all basal cells equally susceptible and permissive for the early events of the viral life cycle or is this a property of a subset only of the basal cell population? The early work of LaPorta and Taichmann (1982) would suggest that virus entry to keratinocytes is not restricted to a subset of the population since HPV-1 virions infect foreskin keratinocytes in monolayer culture, but the episome is not stably maintained in these cells. Intuitively one suspects that a virus which is a 'hitch-hiker' in the keratinocyte in its journey from basal cell to squame gets in at the very beginning of the ride and that the cell permissive for the early events of the viral life cycle is a primitive cell in the keratinocyte lineage, probably a stem cell.

There is some evidence to a support this speculation and perhaps the most persuasive data comes from the rabbit model, where the available information suggests that only keratinocytes migrating from the hair follicle after wounding are infectable (reviewed in Kreider and Bartlett 1981). Thus CRPV induced papillomas develop only on hair-bearing skin; wounding of hair-bearing skin is absolutely required for CRPV infection and importantly the rate of growth of CRPV-induced papillomas is accelerated if the skin is infected during the anagen (active) phase of the hair growth cycle and retarded if the skin is infected during the telogen (inactive) phase. There is now very good evidence that in hair-bearing skin, cells with the characteristics of stem cells, slow-cycling LRC, are present in two sites, the interfollicular epidermis in the centre of the EPU and in the outer root sheath of the hair follicle, an area called the bulge zone (Miller *et al.* 1993). These bulge cells are normally slow cycling but can undergo a transient phase of cell proliferation during early anagen and also after wounding. The LRC of the bulge is a pluripotential cell, capable of regenerating not only the hair follicle but also sebaceous glands and epidermis. In non-hair-bearing skin such as the tongue and vagina, LRC are situated in the basal layer at the tips of the rete pegs in intimate contact with the papillary dermis (Hume and Potten 1983). The sites of putative stem cells in the human cervix are not so clearly identified. Rodent models are not particularly appropriate here since the anatomy and neuro-endocrine control of the rodent genital tract differs considerably from the higher primates. However, as far as analogies can be taken single cells with the features of stem cells occur and are sited at discrete intervals in the basal layer of the squamous epithelium of the cervix. The reserve cell is a pluripotential cell in the sense that it can undergo both glandular and squamous differentiation but the lineage regulation in these cells is unknown.

There are other indirect observations which support the notion that a stem cell is the target cell for infection. There is the interesting phenomenon of the lag phase of several weeks between infection and the first detection of viral activity seen in the rabbit (Kreider and Bartlett 1981) and for which there is anecdotal evidence in humans (Oriel 1971). In the HPV-11 infectious cycle in the nude mouse xenograft model this lag phase is 3–4 weeks and during this time no viral activity can be detected (Stoler *et al.* 1990). An attractive explanation for this would be that the virus infects a stem cell with a long cycle time and the 3–4 week delay is a reflection of the time required for the progeny cells to enter the transit cycling population of the epithelium permissive for transcription of the early region of the genome. Furthermore, a functional mesenchyme or connective tissue is essential for CRPV infection (Breedis and Kreider 1970) and self-renewal in epidermis is exquisitely dependent upon the connective tissue matrix supporting the keratinocyte (Leary *et al.* 1992). Relating to this is the recent and fascinating data from Bossens *et al.* (1992); these workers infected foreskin keratinocytes *in vitro* with caesium-chloride-purified HPV-1 virions obtained from plantar warts and the infected keratinocytes were then grown in organotypic culture using as the matrix de-epidermized human dermis. In this skin-equivalent system amplification of viral DNA could be shown in the reconstituted epidermis and in squames shed from it. In the context of the present discussion it is of interest that in this system good epidermal reconstruction and evidence of viral DNA amplification were found only in the dermal invaginations which are presumptive remnants of hair follicles and exactly the sites where the connective tissue matrix or niche for stem cells might be retained. If this hypothesis that the cell permissive for infection and immediate early viral functions is the stem cell is substantiated it may well turn out that the observed predilection of the HPVs for cutaneous or mucosal surfaces reflects differences in the transcriptional milieu of the stem cell of hair-bearing surfaces compared to mucosal surfaces.

6.6 Virus–keratinocyte interactions at the squamocolumnar junction

The cervix, which appears to be the major site of infection for HPV 16, consists of two epithelial surfaces. The anterior and posterior lips of the vaginal cervix (the ectocervix) are covered by a stratified squamous epithelium similar to that of the vagina. The endocervical canal is lined with tall cylindrical mucous-secreting cells with a characteristic picket fence appearance, interspersed between which are ciliated cells. Between the columnar cells and the basement membrane are small triangular subcolumnar cells. This epithelium lines both the surface and the so-called glands of the endocervix which are in fact a complex system of pits and clefts rather than true racemose glands. The transition between these two epithelia is at the squamocolumnar junction. This junction can be abrupt but more frequently is observed to be a gradual transition between the two types of epithelium, giving rise to a transitional area of cellular instability referred to as the transitional zone. At certain critical physiological periods, principally the late fetal, peri-menarchal, and at the time of first pregnancy the cells at this junction can and do undergo a process described as squamous metaplasia in which simple epithelium is replaced by epithelia with many of the features of stratified squamous epithelium (see Chapter 1). The majority of early neoplastic cervical lesions are located in and around the transformation zone and this has led to the belief that neoplastic change in the cervix occurs as a result of the action of oncogenic agents on metaplastic epithelium resulting in a transformation event.

It is now clear that infection with certain HPVs, in particular HPV 16, 18 and related sub-types, is the major risk factor for the development of cervical neoplasia (Schiffmann 1992). However, HPV 16 in particular is a ubiquitous virus and infects sites in the genital tract such as the penis and anogenital skin (Koutsky *et al.* 1990) but, in comparison to carcinoma of the cervix, carcinoma of the penis and vulva are rare diseases. There are probably several reasons for this but one inference is that the target cell for infection may be crucial in terms of neoplastic transformation and that the metaplastic cell is more susceptible to HPV-mediated transformation than the normal cervical keratinocyte. A central question to address therefore is does the infectious cycle of HPV differ in the metaplastic cell as compared to the normal ectocervical keratinocyte? Addressing this issue requires some understanding of the lineage and differentiation programme of both cell types—information which is rudimentary.

The progenitor cell for metaplastic cervical epithelium is considered to be the reserve cell of the endocervix. There is quite good evidence now that this thesis is correct from animal models (Darwiche *et al.* 1993) and from studies on the histogenesis of metaplastic epithelium using keratin polypeptide expression as markers of cell lineage and differentiation. Squamous cervical metaplasia expresses a unique set of cytokeratin polypeptides (Gigi Leitner *et al.* 1986) which comprise keratins characteristic of simple epithelia—8 and 18—as well as those of the ectocervix—19, 4, 13, and 14. The keratin profile of the reserve cell is somewhat contentious. In a study using chain-specific monoclonal antibodies (M Abs) Levy *et al.* (1988) concluded that there were at least four cell types residing in the endocervix; columnar non-ciliated cells, ciliated cells, and two sub-populations of reserve cells. One of these sub-populations expressed K13, usually a marker of differentiation in cervical squamous epithelium. On the basis of these observations they proposed that metaplastic squamous epithelium derived from a K13 positive reserve cell population. However, Smedts *et al.* (1990) could not identify K13 in reserve cells. Recently (Smedts *et al.* 1992) these workers, using a panel of chain-specific M Abs for keratins 5, 14, and 17, have provided persuasive evidence that the expression of K17 characterizes both immature and mature squamous metaplasia and is expressed consistently in reserve cells. In this study K17 was expressed sporadically in squamous intra-epithelial lesions but progression of CINs was accompanied by an increase in the intensity of staining for K13 and 50 per cent of CIN III in this study were positive for K17. Since most carcinomas studied to date are K17 positive this led these authors to speculate that K17 positive CIN may represent a subset of progressive lesions. The pattern of expression of K17 in epithelia in general is interesting since it strongly depends upon cell position (Troyanovsky *et al.* 1989) with specific expression in basal cells in transitional epithelium and myo-epithelial cells in complex epithelia. The expression of K17 in normal ectocervical epithelium is sporadic and restricted to the occasional basal cell. The pattern of expression of this keratin warrants further investigation with an extended range of reagents since it may identify a subset of primitive basal cells. In this context it is interesting that normal cervical keratinocytes *in vitro* express K17 consistently at a low level (Dixon, unpublished thesis, 1985).

Permissive growth of HPVs is absolutely dependent upon a complete differentiation programme and this begs the question: does the metaplastic squamous cell undergo complete differentiation? There is no good answer to this since there is little information on the spinous to granular transition and expression of markers of terminal differentiation such as loricrin and filaggrin in metaplasia. However, metaplastic cells do have a keratin intermediate filament network which differs from regular ectocervical epithelium since in the basal and parabasal layers they express the simple epithelial keratins 8 and 18 (Smedts *et al.* 1990). The importance of the keratin cytoskeleton in the regulated expression of the keratinocyte differentiation programme has become clear recently (Vassar *et al.* 1991) with the demonstration that single base mutations in the genes encoding one keratin polypeptide can result in the loss of epithelial integrity. The keratins truly function as a cell skeleton; they provide mechanical strength, control cell shape, and crucially regulate the plasticity of the cell—factors of central importance in the keratinocyte in which movement upward from the basal layer is tightly linked to differentiation. The temporal expression of keratin pairs *in vivo* is very strictly regulated during normal differentiation. Recent studies have made it clear that the expression and assembly of the differentiation-specific keratins of the stratum granulosum is dependent upon the pre-existing intermediate filament network of the basal layers— if this is abnormal, filament assembly in the superficial layers is disrupted (Kartasova *et al.* 1993). In view of these observations it seems quite probable that the metaplastic keratinocyte either does not undergo a normal differentiation programme or fails to complete the lineage or both. Speculatively one could suggest that metaplastic epithelium is only semi-permissive for HPV—the reserve cell is readily infected, permissive for the immediate early events of viral growth and for early region transcription but that the crucial signals for capsid protein synthesis which seem to co-incide with a spinous to granular transition do not take place.

6.7   Implications for immune responses

HPVs are exclusively intra-epithelial pathogens and virus replication is differentiation-dependent and this is of profound importance for host defences to these agents. The most obvious aspect of the infectious cycle is the time taken to complete it. At its most rapid the time taken from infection to viral assembly and release will be 1–2 weeks since this is the minimum time taken for the basal to superficial differentiation. These are very conservative estimates and both experimental data from animal models and clinical observation suggests that the period between infection and the appearance of a lesion is of the order of 6–8 weeks. A key aspect of virus–host interactions must therefore be the ability to evade host defences for quite long periods of time. Clearly HPV does this very successfully since a characteristic of warts and other lesions induced by these agents is persistence over months and years. The mechanisms underlying this evasion of host defences are certainly not understood but the replication cycle may represent a mechanism for this. As far as is known only keratino-cytes are permissive for the immediate early viral functions and although it is possible that HPV can infect many cells, viral proteins are expressed only in keratinocytes and presented to the immune system therefore in the context of the class I of the keratinocyte, a non-professional antigen pre-senting cell. This is a scenario for the induction of peripheral tolerance to these proteins. Furthermore virus infects basal cells at low copy number and viral gene expression is virtually undetectable in the lower layers of the epithelium; high levels of viral gene expression and the production of particles take place only in the terminally differentiated layers far removed from the systemic immune defences. Finally it must be remembered that HPV is not a passive passenger in the keratinocyte but reprogrammes the cell to permit viral replication. The keratinocyte is a key component in the dynamic cellular society of the epithelium in which lymphocytes, macrophages, and Langerhans cells are entering and leaving in a regulated manner, and disruption of this traffic may be an important mechanism by which HPV evades detection.

References

Bedell, M. A., Hudson, J. B., Golub, T. R., Turyk, M. E., Hosken, M., Wilbanks, G. D. *et al.* (1991). Amplification of human papillomavirus genomes *in vitro* is dependent on epithelial differentiation. *Journal of Virology*, **65**, 2254–60.

Bossens, M., Van Pachterbeke, C., Tuynder, M., Parent, D., Heenen, M., and Rommelaere, J. (1992). *in vitro* infection of normal human keratinocytes by human papillomavirus type 1 followed by amplification of the viral genome in reconstructed epidermis. *Journal of General Virology*, **73**, 3269–73.

Breedis, C. and Kreider, J. W. (1970). The role of the dermis in the induction of neoplasia by Shope papilloma virus. *Cancer Research*, **30**, 974–80.

Darwiche, N., Celli, G., Sly, L., Lancillotti, F., and De Luca, L. M. (1993). Retinoid status controls the appearance of reserve cells and keratin expression in mouse cervical epithelium. *Cancer Research*, **53**, 2287–99.

Dixon, I. S. and Stanley, M. A. (1984). Immunofluorescent studies of human cervical epithelia *in vitro* using antibodies against specific keratin components. *Molecular Biology Medicine*, **2**, 37–51.

Dlugosz, A. A. and Yuspa, S. H. (1993). Coordinate changes in gene expression which mark the spinous to granular transition in epidermis are regulated by protein kinase C. *Journal of Cell Biology*, **120**, 217–25.

Dollard, S. C., Broker, T. R., and Chow, L. T. (1993). Regulation of the human papillomavirus type 11 E6 promoter by viral and host transcription factors in primary human keratinocytes. *Journal of Virology*, **67**, 1721–26.

Gigi Leitner, O., Geiger, B., Levy, R., and Czernobilsky, B. (1986). Cytokeratin expression in metaplasia of the human cervix. *Differentiation*, **31**, 191–205.

Higgins, G. D., Phillips, G. E., Smith, L. A., Uzelin, D. M., and Burrell, C. J. (1992). High prevalence of human papillomavirus transcripts in all grades of cervical intra-epithelial glandular neoplasia. *Cancer*, **70**, 136–46.

Hume, W. J. and Potten, C. S. (1983). Proliferative units in stratified squamous epithelium. *Clinical Experiments in Dermatology*, **8**, 93–106.

Hummel, M., Hudson, J. B., and Laimins, L. A. (1992). Differentiation induced and constitutive transcription of human papillomavirus type 31b in cell lines containing viral episomes. *Journal of Virology*, **66**, 6070–80.

Kartasova, T., Roop, D. R., Holbrook, K. A., and Yuspa, S. H. (1993). Mouse differentiation-specific keratins 1 and 10 require a preexisting keratin scaffold to form a network. *Journal of Cell Biology*, **120**, 1251–61.

Kennedy, I. M., Haddow, J. K., and Clements, J. B. (1991). A negative regulatory element in the human papillomavirus type 16 genome acts at the level of late mRNA stability. *Journal of Virology*, **65**, 2093–7.

Koutsky, L. A., Galloway, D. A., and Holmes, K. K. (1988). Epidemiology of genital human papillomavirus infection. *Epidemiologic Review*, **10**, 122–163.

Kreider, J. W. and Bartlett, G. L. (1981). The Shope papilloma-carcinoma complex of rabbits: a model system of neoplastic progression and spontaneous regression. *Advances in Cancer Research*, **35**, 81–110.

Kreider, J. W., Howett, M. K., Wolfe, S. A., Bartlett, G. L., Zaino, R. J., Sedlacek, T. *et al.* (1985). Morphological transformation *in vivo* of human uterine cervix with papillomavirus from condylomata acuminata. *Nature*, **317**, 639–41.

Kreider, J. W., Howett, M. K., Lill, N. L., Bartlett, G. L., Zaino, R. J., Sedlacek, T. V. *et al.* (1986). *in vivo* transformation of human skin with human papillomavirus type 11 from condylomata acuminata. *Journal of Virology*, **59**, 369–76.

LaPorta, R. F. and Taichman, L. B. (1982). Human papilloma viral DNA replicates as a stable episome in cultured epidermal keratinocytes. *Proceedings of the National Academy of Sciences (USA)*, **79**, 3393–7.

Leary, T., Jones, P. L., Appleby, M. W., Blight, A., Parkinson, E. K., and Stanley, M. A. (1992). Epidermal keratinocyte self renewal is dependent upon dermal integrity. *Journal of Investigative Dermatology*, **99**, 422–30.

Levy, R., Czernobilsky, B., and Geiger, B. (1988). Subtyping of epithelial cells of normal and metaplastic human uterine cervix using poly-peptide specific cytokeratin antibodies. *Differentiation*, **39**, 185–95.

Mehrel, T., Hohl, D., Rothnagel, J. A., Longley, M. A., Bundman, D., Cheng, C. *et al.* (1990). Identification of a major keratinocyte cell envelope protein, loricrin. *Cell*, **61**, 1103–12.

Merrick, D. T., Blanton, R. A., Gown, A. M., and McDougall, J. K. (1992). Altered expression of proliferation and differentiation markers in human papillomavirus 16 and 18 immortalized epithelial cells grown in organotypic culture. *American Journal of Pathology*, **140**, 167–77.

Meyer, C., Frattine, M. G., Hudson. J. B., and Laimins, L. A. (1992). Biosynthesis of human papillomavirus from a continuous cell line upon epithelial differentiation. *Science*, **257**, 1131–42.

Miller, S. J., Sun, T., and Lavker, R. M. (1993). Hair follicles, stem cells and skin cancer. *Journal of Investigative Dermatology*, **100**, 289s–94s.

Moll, R., Franke, W. W., Schiller, D. L., Geiger, B., and Krepler, R. (1982). The catalog of human cytokeratins: patterns of expression in normal epithelia, tumors and cultured cells. *Cell*, **31**, 11–24.

Morris, R. J., Fischer, S. M., and Slaga, T. J. (1985). Evidence that the centrally and peripherally located cells in the murine epidermal proliferative unit are two distinct populations. *Journal of Investigative Dermatology*, **84**, 277–81.

Mungal, S., Steinberg, B. M., and Taichman, L. B. (1992). Replication of plasmid derived human papillomavirus type 11 DNA in cultured keratinocytes. *Journal of Virology*, **66**, 3220–4.

Nelson, W. and Sun, T. (1983). The 50 and 58K dalton keratin classes as molecular markers for stratified squamous epithelia: cell culture studies. *Journal of Cell Biology*, **97**, 244–51.

Oriel, J. D. (1971). Anal warts and anal coitus. *British Journal of Venereal Diseases*, **47**, 373–6.

Polakowska, R. R. and Goldsmith, L. A. (1991). The cell envelope and transglutaminases. In *Physiology, biochemistry and molecular biology of the skin*. (ed. L. A. Goldsmith), pp. 168–201. Oxford University Press, New York.

Potten, C. S. (1974). The epidermal proliferative unit: the possible role of the central basal cell. *Cell Tissue Kinet*, **7**, 77–86.

Rheinwald, J. G. and Green, H. (1975). Serial cultivation of strains of human epidermal keratinocytes: the formation of keratinising colonies from single cells. *Cell*, **6**, 331–44.

Rice, R. H. and Green, H. (1979). Presence in human cells of a soluble precursor of the cross-linked envelope: activation of crosslinking by calcium ions. *Cell*, **18**, 681–94.

Rothnagel, J. A. and Steinert, P. M. (1990). The structure of the gene for filaggrin and a comparison of the repeating units. *Journal of Biological Chemistry*, **265**, 1862–5.

Schiffman, M. H. (1992). Recent progress in defining the epidemiology of human papillomavirus infection and cervical neoplasia. *Journal of the National Cancer Institute*, **84**, 394–8.

Smedts, F., Ramaekers, R., Robben, H., Pruszczynski, M., van Muijen, G., Lane, B. *et al.* (1990). Changing patterns of keratin expression during progression of cervical intra-epithelial neoplasia. *American Journal of Pathology*, **136**, 657–68.

Smedts, F., Ramaekers, F., Troyanovsky, S., Pruszczynski, M., Robben, H., Lane, B. *et al.* (1992). Basal cell keratins in cervical reserve cells and a comparison to their expression in cervical intra-epithelial neoplasia. *American Journal of Pathology*, **140**, 610–12.

Stanley, M. A., Browne, H. M., Appleby, M., and Minson, A. C. (1989). Properties of a non tumorigenic human cervical keratinocyte cell line. *International Journal of Cancer*, **43**, 672–6.

Sterling, J., Stanley, M., Gatward, G., and Minson, T. (1990). Production of human papillomavirus type 16 virions in a keratinocyte cell line. *Journal of Virology*, **64**, 6305–7.

Sterling, J. C., Skepper, J., and Stanley, M. A. (1993). Immunoelectronmicroscopic localisation of HPV 16 L1 and E4 proteins in cervical keratinocytes-cultured *in vivo*. *Journal of Investigative Dermatology*, **100**, 154–58.

Stoler, M. H. and Broker, T. R. (1986). In situ hybridization detection of human papillomavirus DNAs and messenger RNAs in genital condylomas and a cervical carcinoma. *Human Pathology*, **17**, 1250–8.

Stoler, A., Kopan, R., Duvic, M., and Fuchs, E. (1988). Use of monospecific antisera and cDNA probes to localise the major changes in keratin expression during normal and abnormal epidermal differentiation. *Journal of Cell Biology*, **107**, 427–446.

Stoler, M. H., Wolinsky, S. M., Whitbeck, A., Broker, T. R., and Chow, L. T. (1989). Differentiation linked human papillomavirus types 6 and 11 transcription in genital condylomata revealed by in situ hybridization with message specific RNA probes. *Virology*, **172**, 331–40.

Stoler, M. H., Whitbeck, A., Wolinsky, S. M., Broker, T. R., Chow, L. T., Howett, M. K. *et al.* (1990). Infectious cycle of human papillomavirus type 11 in human foreskin xenografts in nude mice. *Journal of Virology*, **64**, 3310–18.

Stoler, M. H., Rhodes, C. R., Whitbeck, A., Wolinsky, S. M., Chow, L. T., and Broker, T. R. (1992). Human papillomavirus type 16 and 18 gene expression in cervical neoplasias. *Human Pathology*, **23**, 117–28.

Troyanovsky, S. M., Guelstein, T. A., Krutovskikh, V. H., and Bannikov, G. A. (1989). Patterns of expression of K17 in human epithelia: dependency on cell position. *Journal of Cell Science*, **93**, 419–26.

Vassar, R., Coulombe, P. A., Degenstein, L., Albers, K., and Fuchs, E. (1991). Mutant keratin expression in transgenic mice causes marked abnormalities resembling a human genetic skin disease. *Cell*, **64**, 365–80.

Weber, B., Horiguchi, J., Luebbers, R., Sherman, M., and Kufe, D. (1989). Post-transcriptional stabilization of c-fms mRNA by a labile protein during human monocytic differentiation. *Molecular Cell Biology*, **9**, 769–75.

Zhu, Y., Schwartz, R. J., and Crow, M. T. (1991). Phorbol esters selectively downregulate contractile protein expression in terminally differentiated myotubes through transcriptional repression and message destabilization. *Journal of Cell Biology*, **115**, 745–54.

7 Serological immune response to HPV

LUTZ GISSMANN and MARTIN MULLER

7.1 Introduction

Diagnosis of viral infections can be performed by analysing the specimen from the patient either for the presence of the infectious agent (e.g. by infection and growth of the agent *in vitro*) or by identification of the genome or expression of the genes of the pathogen, that is, the genetic material (by nucleic acid hybridization) or one of the viral proteins (eg. by ELISA). This approach is usually successful during the acute phase of a disease but may fail during the unapparent intermission of an infection as in this situation virus production is usually very low and the test may be negative due to sampling problems. In the case of human papillomaviruses, particularly those which affect the anogenital mucosa, persistent infection without clinical symptoms is a rather common phenomenon (see Chapter 1).

In contrast to the detection of the infectious agent, the humoral immune response which develops as a consequence of the exposure of the host to the virus usually can be measured life-long although antibody titres may drop to levels below detection after time. Measuring the humoral immune response is not only relevant in order to diagnose certain virus-induced diseases which are of clinical importance such as hepatitis B, measles, or rubella, but also provides important information about the development of antibodies directed against the individual viral proteins which appear as the infection proceeds. Thus serology is an important tool in the study of the natural history of viral infections. This aspect is of particular relevance in the case of those viruses which are able to persist within the infected tissue such as hepatitis B virus or members of the herpes virus group (e.g. Epstein–Barr virus) as well as the papillomaviruses. In addition, a profound knowledge about the natural history of an infection is critical for the design of vaccination strategies against the etiologic agent.

7.2 Preparation of viral antigens

Most of the clinically relevant viruses can be grown in experimental systems such as animal cell cultures, and the viral antigens required for the detection of specific antibodies in human sera can easily be prepared. Thus, virus particles can be harvested from infected cells and used after purification to measure the response to the structural (late) proteins. Viral proteins which are not packaged into particles but provide vital functions for the virus' life cycle such as the replication of the viral nucleic acid ('early' proteins) cannot easily be obtained. In such cases, the infected cell *per se* can be used as source of antigen for certain serological tests performed *in situ* such as immunofluorescence. In fact, for many viral infections the humoral immune response has been characterized by the use of such 'authentic' antigens before 'synthetic' proteins produced by recombinant DNA technology using a variety of systems became available.

During the last few years, substantial progress has been made towards the development of techniques for papillomavirus replication under laboratory conditions (see Chapter 6). Up to the present time, however, permissive papillomavirus growth in experimental systems cannot yield the quantities of virus which are required for the preparation of antigens to be used in routine serological assays. On the other hand, replication of the mucosotropic human papillomaviruses in clinical lesions is very limited, too. Thus neither the early nor the late viral proteins are easily available for use as antigens in serological assays. As an exception, human papillomavirus type II can be amplified to a certain extent in human epithelium which has been infected *in vitro* and is transplanted into immunocompromised mice (Kreider *et al.* 1987). Particles obtained from this system have been used to measure antibodies against HPV II late proteins (Bonnez *et al.* 1991, 1992; see below).

In general, for use in serological assays papillomavirus proteins or parts thereof are expressed using a variety of prokaryotic and eukaryotic recombinant vectors in different hosts such as *E. coli*, yeast, baculovirus/insect cells, or vaccinia virus/animal cells (Table 7.1). Under experimental conditions the individual systems have been shown to have different advantages and disadvantages. Thus, the *bacterial vectors* usually produce high quantities of the viral proteins which, however, are not modified (e.g. glycosylated) post-translationally as in the natural infection. In addition, eukaryotic proteins may often be unstable in bacteria unless they are linked to a prokaryotic peptide such as, for example, the bacterial beta-galactosidase). Such fusion proteins can easily be used when antibodies to linear epitopes (Fig. 7.1) are to be measured (e.g. in Western blot assay; see below). They are certainly less well suited for the detection of antibodies directed against conformational epitopes (Fig. 7.1) since the three-dimensional structure of the protein may be influenced by the heterologous peptide fused to it. The *eukaryotic viral vectors*, on the other hand, supposedly provide the authentic proteins but often at lower yields as compared to the bacterial systems, mainly because the infected cells can be grown to large quantities only in industrial settings. Such systems, however,

Table 7.1 Methods used for the detection of HPV-specific antibodies in human sera

	Antigen	Origin of antigen	Advantages	Disadvantages
ELISA	Peptides	Chemically synthesized	Feasibility	Linear epitopes
	Proteins	E. coli, yeast	Conformational epitopes	Purification required
	Virus particles	Infected human tissue	Authentic antigen	Antigen is difficult to prepare
Western blotting	Fusion proteins	E. coli	False positive reaction can be identified	Tedious
RIPA	Protein	In vitro transcribed/translated	Conformational epitopes, high sensitivity	Tedious
Immunofluorescence	Protein	Eukaryotic vector	Modification of protein, conformational epitopes	Low sensitivity

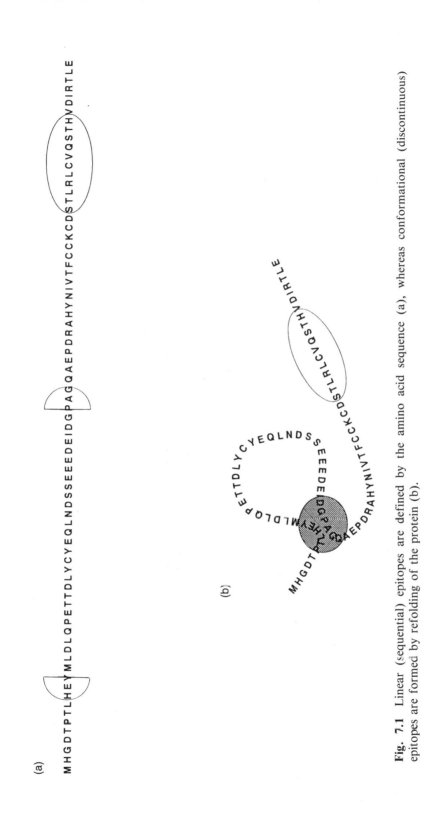

Fig. 7.1 Linear (sequential) epitopes are defined by the amino acid sequence (a), whereas conformational (discontinuous) epitopes are formed by refolding of the protein (b).

may prove very useful for the characterization of the cellular localization of the viral protein (Zhou *et al.* 1991) as measured by *in situ* techniques such as immunofluorescence using specific antisera experimentally produced in animals. This approach is also feasible for the detection of antibodies in human sera (Nindl and Gissmann, unpublished data) but its sensitivity and specificity in comparison to other assays still needs to be investigated. Eukaryotic viral vector systems certainly are the ideal tools to study cellular immune responses (see Chapter 8). Since yeast is an eukaryotic organism that can easily be grown to high titres even under laboratory conditions it should provide the properly modified protein in combination with a high yield of expression when appropriate vectors are used (Tommasino *et al.* 1990; Carter *et al.* 1991).

Proteins which are expressed by one of the recombinant vectors can either be used as antigens for the detection of antibodies as discussed below or, alternatively, expression of parts of proteins can be used as a tool to identify seroreactive regions (Muller *et al.* 1990). Identification of such regions is necessary when type-specific reagents need to be prepared or when synthetic peptides are to be used as antigens. Synthetic peptides produced in an analytical scale have also proved suitable for the definition of seroreactive regions (Dillner 1990; Suchankova *et al.* 1992). A compilation of epitopes used by different investigators was published recently (Viscidi and Shah 1992).

7.3   Principles of serological assays

Most of the assays which are used in modern viral serodiagnostics are based upon direct measurement of the antigen–antibody interaction, e.g. radio-immunoassay (RIA), enzyme-linked immunosorbent assay (ELISA), Western blotting (WB), or immuno-fluorescence. For the detection of HPV-specific antibodies in human sera mostly WB or ELISA have been used. The *Western blotting* technique (Fig. 7.2) is a time-consuming, labour-intensive procedure and has proved to be unsuitable for the screening of large serum collections. It is based on the electrophoresis of the protein under denaturing conditions through SDS-polyacrylamide gels followed by transfer to a membrane. The membrane is incubated with the sample to be tested and if antibodies became bound to the protein they are visualized by enzyme-coupled secondary antibodies which are specific for human gamma-globulin. The membrane is finally incubated with a suitable substrate for the enzyme which induces a colour reaction at the position where the reactive protein was banded.

Thus the WB technique enables the identification of a specific reaction even if the protein was not completely purified prior to the electrophoresis. The strength of the reaction correlates to the amount of reactive antibodies

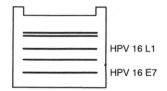

Separation of the proteins by SDS-
polyacrylamide gel electrophoresis

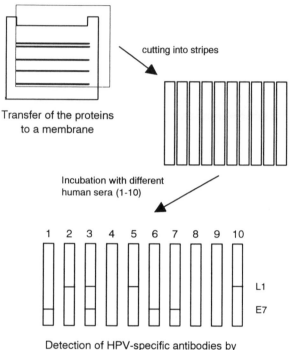

Transfer of the proteins
to a membrane

cutting into stripes

Incubation with different
human sera (1-10)

Detection of HPV-specific antibodies by
incubation with enzyme-labelled second
antibody and staining with substrate

Fig. 7.2 Detection of antibodies in human sera by Western blotting. Specific reaction can be identified even if the antigen preparation contains some protein contamination.

which were present in the sample but it can be monitored only in a semi-quantitative manner. On the other hand, by this assay antibodies to sequential (linear) rather than discontinuous (conformational) epitopes are measured since the protein is bound to the membrane in a more or less denatured form. Enzyme-linked secondary antibodies are also used in

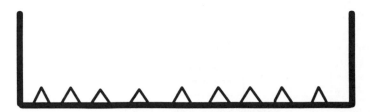

Coating a microtitre plate with the antigen under study

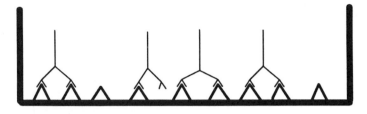

Testing sera for antibodies reactive with the antigen

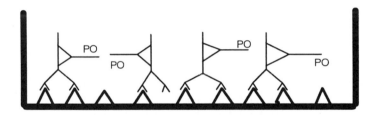

Reaction of the human antibodies with enzyme-,
e.g. peroxidase (PO)- labelled second antibodies

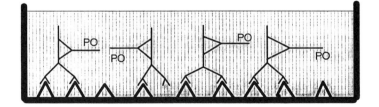

Addition of substrate to observe colour change

Fig. 7.3   Detection of human antibodies by ELISA.

ELISAs (Fig. 7.3) to monitor the antigen–antibody reaction. Since in this case the intensity of the colour reaction is measured photometrically, the amount of the antibodies bound to the antigen can be quantified. The antigen is loaded into the wells of a microtitre plate, and all reactions are carried out in a small volume. By ELISA many samples can be tested at the same time and the processing is partly automated, thus this assay is well suited for routine screening of serum samples. Either synthetic peptides derived from the individual proteins (see above), whole proteins, or complete virus particles have been used as antigens. Synthetic peptides represent well-defined reagents as they can be efficiently purified by high-performance liquid chromatography (HPLC). This procedure eliminates the risk of false positive results due to cross-reactions with contaminating non-viral products such as bacterial cell components when fusion proteins made in *E. coli* are applied. As the whole HPV proteins may consist of type-specific as well as of papillomavirus-common epitopes, synthetic peptides may be preferable in certain instances. On the other hand, antibodies directed against conformational epitopes are very likely not to be detected by synthetic peptides. It is anticipated that the use of native proteins may reduce the number of false negative samples although a careful validation by comparison of different antigens still needs to be done.

In contrast to the direct measurement of antigen–antibody complexes as discussed above, their detection can be based upon changes in the physicochemical or biological properties of the antigen which are induced by the interaction with the antibody. Thus the infectivity of a virus may be reduced if it is covered by (neutralizing) antibodies. The reduction of infectivity can be quantified (by neutralization assay) and is taken as a direct correlate for the amount of antibody present in a given serum specimen. *Neutralization* of infectious HPV II particles was demonstrated recently with sera from patients with condylomata acuminata (Christensen *et al.* 1991). The method of heterotransplantation of infected human epithelium (Kreider *et al.* 1987) which was used in this study is too tedious to be useful for quantification of antibodies by testing serial serum dilutions and certainly cannot be used for routine screening of serum samples. Recently, *radio-immunoprecipitation* (RIPA) (Fig. 7.4) was introduced for the detection of HPV-specific antibodies (Muller *et al.* 1992). This method takes advantage of the fact that antigen–antibody complexes can easily be precipitated when they react with protein A of *Staphylococcus aureus* or with a secondary antibody coupled to a carrier such as sepharose. The precipitate is subsequently dissociated and separated on an SDS polyacrylamide gel. When radioactively labelled viral protein (in case of HPV produced by an *in vitro* transcription/translation protocol) is used for the reaction with the antibodies it can be monitored with high sensitivity by autoradiography and thus demonstrates the presence of specific antibodies within the particular sample. Since the complete protein is used, antibodies recognizing conformational epitopes should be detected by RIPA.

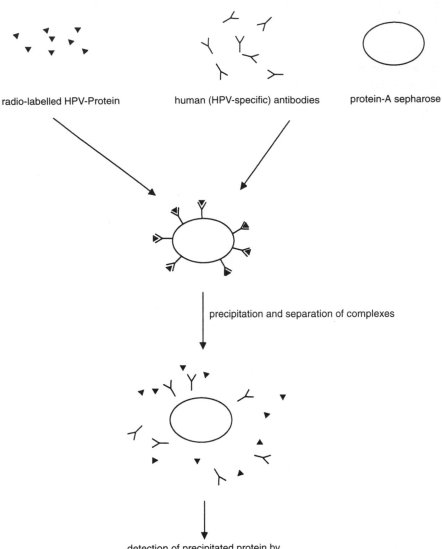

radio-labelled HPV-Protein   human (HPV-specific) antibodies   protein-A sepharose

precipitation and separation of complexes

detection of precipitated protein by
SDS-gel electrophoresis and autoradiography

Fig. 7.4 Detection of human antibodies by radio-immunoprecipitation. The detection of the labelled viral protein depends on the presence of antibodies prior to precipitation.

This assay, however, gives only semiquantitative results and is too time-consuming to be useful for routine testing.

7.4   Type-specificity of individual assays

The immune response to papillomaviruses in general is not expected to be very pronounced since they do not get into such an intimate contact with the immune system in comparison with those viruses in which a viremia occurs during the course of their replication. In fact, the production of papillomaviruses is restricted to the differentiating part of the epithelium and synthesis of virus structural proteins and assembly of particles occurs within the superficial layers. In the case of human papillomaviruses which infect the anogenital tract, virus production is very low. In view of the fact that among the members of the papillomavirus family there is considerable amino acid homology within the late proteins L1 and L2 (see Chapter 2), it is not clear whether the antibodies directed against the late proteins which can be measured by different methods (see below) are actually HPV type-specific although within the L2 protein type-specific epitopes have been shown to exist (Jenison *et al.* 1991). It is conceivable that there exist different populations of cross-reacting antibodies which have developed as a response to infections with other human papillomaviruses, in particular the efficiently replicating HPV types such as HPV 1 which is responsible for the induction of common warts.

The early viral proteins (e.g. E2, E6, and E7) which are expressed in the deeper layers of the infected epithelium are not produced to high quantities but surprisingly high antibody titres are measured in some sera obtained from cervical cancer patients. The occurrence of cross-reacting antibodies cannot, of course, be excluded in all instances, but at least for HPV 16 and HPV 18 the detection of antibodies to the E6 and E7 proteins appears to be type-specific since a good correlation between the presence of HPV 16 and HPV 18 DNA within a patient's cervical cancer biopsy and the reactivity of the corresponding serum has been demonstrated (Bleul *et al.* 1991; Muller *et al.* 1992). A strong antibody response may also be explained by the long persistence of HPV-positive and protein-expressing lesions which eventually may lead to cervical cancer. Alternatively, viral proteins may be released from cancer cells due to cell death and necrosis of the tumour. In fact, preliminary data indicate that antibody titres against E6 or E7 rise as a consequence of the tumour size (Gissmann *et al.* unpublished data).

In terms of quantity and localization of expression, the protein E4 seems to have an intermediate position between the typical early proteins and the structural proteins. In parallel with other early proteins, E4 is expressed in the intermediate and spinous layers of the epithelium but the level of its production is even higher than that observed for the late proteins. In fact, the level of antibodies directed against the E4 protein can also mount to high titres. As has been discussed above the question of cross-reactivity of antibodies which have developed as a consequence of infection with other papillomavirus types cannot be ignored but the problem of false positive results appears unlikely since, among the different HPV types, the E4 open reading frame represents one of the least conserved regions of the whole genome. There are some discrepancies reported in the literature when antibody prevalences are measured either with different synthetic peptides or with complete proteins (see below) and the specificity of the different reagents still has to be evaluated.

7.5   Humoral immune response to human papillomaviruses associated with anogenital lesions

Before the introduction of recombinant DNA technology, studies on the immune response against papillomavirus infections were mostly restricted to those HPV types which induce the development of skin warts such as verrucae vulgares (for review see Spradbrow 1987) because, in comparison to the mucosotropic HPV types, the virus replication within those lesions is much more efficient. Recent studies, which are discussed below, deal almost exclusively with the characterization of the humoral immune response to the HPV types 6, 11, 16, and 18. The majority of publications present data on the presence of antibodies of the IgG class and some information is available on the IgA response.

7.6   Antibodies as marker for HPV-associated diseases

Antibodies to late viral proteins of HPV 6 or HPV 11 are found to be predominant in patients suffering from *condylomata acuminata* or in children with recurrent *respiratory papillomatosis* (Suchankova *et al.* 1990; Bonnez *et al.* 1991, 1992) conditions caused almost exclusively by these viral types. This is not an unexpected finding since within these lesions there is reasonably efficient virus replication and antibodies directed against the structural proteins may develop as a consequence of reinfection when, after damage of the epithelium, the virus comes into contact with the basal cells of the epithelium. Interestingly, the most remarkable differences between patients and healthy controls were measured when complete HPV 11 virus particles were used, although a significant proportion of patients failed to react. In contrast, with synthetic peptides some reactivity was also seen in sera obtained from asymptomatic individuals. In fact, in some studies applying bacterial fusion proteins no differences at all were found between cases and controls (for review see Viscidi and Shah 1992). Towards this end, it is unclear whether linear epitopes as they are present in Western blot assays or ELISAs are more sensitive reagents and thus also react in individuals with a history of clinical lesions or with subclinical papilloma-virus infections. Alternatively some of the linear epitopes may be cross-reacting with antibodies directed against the corresponding proteins of other papillomavirus types.

The occurrence of HPV-specific antibodies in patients with intra-epi-thelial lesions of the anogenital region which are mostly associated with HPV 16 (see Chapter 1) is still controversial, and serological markers for the precursor lesions of cervical cancer have not yet been identified. Thus, a specific association of E4-specific antibodies with STD patients or with women who were referred to a colposcopy clinic because of an abnormal PAP smear was found by Western blot analysis and by peptide-ELISA (Jochmus-Kudielka *et al.* 1989); Muller *et al.* 1993) but this finding was not confirmed by other investigators (Suchankova *et al.* 1992). In con-trast, the presence of HPV 16 E4-specific antibodies in cervical cancer patients which, although only seen in a small proportion of the samples, was statistically significant in comparison to age-matched controls (Kochel *et al.* 1991; Kanda *et al.* 1992). Since the first report published in 1989, the correlation of E7-specific antibodies with HPV 16 or HPV 18 positive cervical cancer has been confirmed by using different methods for antibody detection including ELISA and radio-immunoprecipitation and is now well established in the literature (reviewed by Viscidi and Shah 1992; Muller *et al.* 1992; Kanda *et al.* 1992). A similar association was also found for E6-specific antibodies (Muller *et al.* 1992; Nindl and Gissmann, unpublished data) but this finding still needs to be confirmed in further studies. Sur-prisingly, antibodies to both E6 and E7 are found in only up to 50–70 per cent of sera obtained from cervical cancer patients with proven HPV 16- or HPV 18-positive cancer biopsies. It is unclear why certain patients fail to develop antibodies and possible explanations will be discussed else-where (Gissmann 1993).

7.7   Serology as a tool to study the natural history of genital HPV infections

Infection with genital papillomaviruses can lead to the induction of overt lesions but also, and very likely in the majority of cases, to the establish-ment of unapparent viral persistence within the epithelium without de-velopment of macroscopically visible disease. It is not clear whether the outcome of an infection is determined at the outset of the infection and which factors influence this or to what extent the virus can switch between the latent and active state. Follow-up of individuals by serological assays may be a helpful tool to investigate these questions which are critical for an understanding of the biology of papillomaviruses. In some instances, however, the specificity of the available assays has not yet been validated by comparison to the clinical picture (i.e. the presence of a lesion in sero-positive patients) or to the detection of specific HPV DNA within the patient's sample. Antibodies to HPV 16 proteins have been found in a considerable proportion of young children (Jenison *et al.* 1990; Muller and Gissmann, unpublished data; Vonka, personal communication). The significance of this finding remains unclear and it has to be investigated whether in these samples cross-reacting antibodies were detected or whether infection with HPV 16 actually occurs frequently at young age and can be transmitted via a non-sexual route.

References

Bleul, C., Muller, M., Frank, R., Gausepohl, H., Koldovsky, U., Mgaya, H. N. *et al.* (1991). Human papillomavirus type 18 E6 and E7 antibodies in human sera: increased anti-E7 prevalence in cervical and cancer patients. *Journal of Clinical Microbiology*, **29**, 1579–88.

Bonnez, W., Da-Rin, C., Rose, R. C., and Reichman, R. C. (1991). Use of human papillomavirus type II virions in an ELISA to detect specific antibodies in humans with *condylomata acuminata*. *Journal of General Virology*, **72**, 1343–7.

Bonnez, W., Kashima, H. K., Leventhal, B., Mounts, P., Rose, R. C., Reichman, R. C. *et al.* (1992). Antibody response to human papillomavirus (HPV) type II in children with juvenile-onset recurrent respiratory papillomatosis (RRP). *Virology*, **188**, 384–7.

Carter, J. J., Yaegashi, N., Jenison, S. A., and Galloway, D. A. (1991). Expression of human papillomavirus proteins in yeast saccharomyces cerevisiae. *Virology*, **182**, 513–21.

Christensen, N. D., Kreider, J. W., Shah, K. V., and Rando, R. F. (1992). Detection of human serum antibodies that neutralize infectious human papilloma-virus type II virions. *Journal of General Virology*, **73**, 1261–7.

Dillner, J. (1990). Mapping of linear epitopes of human papillomavirus type 16: the E1, E2, E3, E4, E5, E6 and E7 open reading frames. *International Journal of Cancer*, **46**, 703–11.

Gissmann, L. (1993). The current role of HPV serology. In *Human papillomavirus infections in dermatovenereology* (ed. G. Gross and G. von Krogh), CRC Press, Boca Raton, in preparation.

Jenison, S. A., Yu, X.-P., Valentine, J. M., Koutsky, L. A., Christiansen, A. E., Beckmann, A. M. *et al.* (1990). Evidence of prevalent genital-type human papil-lomavirus infections in adults and children. *Journal of Infectious Disease*, **162**, 60–9.

Jenison, S. A., Yu, X.-P., Valentine, J. M., Koutsky, L. A., Christiansen, A. E., Beckmann, A. M. *et al.* (1991). Characterization of human antibody-reactive epitopes encoded by human papillomavirus types 16 and 18. *Journal of Virology*, **65**, 1208–18.

Jochmus-Kudielka, I., Schneider, A., Braun, R., Kimmig, R., Koldovsky, U., Schneweis, K. E. *et al.* (1989). Antibodies against the human papillomavirus type 16 early proteins in human sera: correlation of anti-E7 reactivity and cervical cancer. *Journal of the National Cancer Institute*, **81**, 1698–704.

Kanda, T., Onda, T., Zanma, S., Yasugi, T., Furuno, A., Watanabe, S. *et al.* (1992). Independent association of antibodies against human papillomavirus type 16 E1/E4 and E7 proteins with cervical cancer. *Virology*, **190**, 724–32.

Kochel, H. G., Monazahian, M., Sievert, K., Hoehne, M., Thomssen, C., Teichmann, A. *et al.* (1991). Occurrence of antibodies to L1, L2, E4 and E7 gene products of human papillomavirus types 6b, 16 and 18 among cervical cancer patients and controls. *International Journal of Cancer*, **48**, 682–8.

Kreider, J. W., Howett, M. K., Leure-Dupree, A. E., Zaino, R. J., and Weber, J. A. (1987). Laboratory production of infectious human papillomavirus type II. *Journal of Virology*, **61**, 590–3.

Muller, M., Gausepohl, H., de Martynoff, G., Frank, R., Brasseur, R., and Gissmann, L. (1990). Identification of seroreactive regions of the human papillomavirus type 16 protein E4, E6, E7 and L1. *Journal of General Virology*, **71**, 2709–17.

Muller, M., Viscidi, R. P., Sun, Y., Guerrero, E., Hill, P. M., Shah, F. *et al.* (1992). Antibodies to HPV 16 E6 and E7 proteins as markers for HPV 16-associated invasive cervical cancer. *Virology*, **187**, 508–14.

Spradbrow, P. B. (1987). Immune response to papillomavirus infection. In *Papillomaviruses and human disease* (ed. K. Syrjaenen, L. Gissmann and L. G. Koss), pp. 334–70. Springer-Verlag, Berlin.

Suchankova, A., Ritter, O., Hirsch, I., Krchnak, V., Vagner, J., Kalos, Z. *et al.* (1990). Presence of antibody reactive with synthetic peptide derived from L2 open reading frame of human papillomavirus types 6b and 11 in human sera. *Acta Virology*, **34**, 433–42.

Suchankova, A., Krchnak, V., Vagner, J., Krcmar, M., Ritterova, L., and Vonka, V. (1992). Epitope mapping of the human papillomavirus type 16 E4 protein by synthetic peptides. *Journal of General Virology*, **73**, 429–32.

Tommasino, M., Contorni, M., Scarlato, V., Bugnoli, M., Maundrell, K., and Cavalieri, F. (1990). Synthesis, phosphorylation and nuclear localization of human papillomavirus E7 protein in *Schizosaccharomyces pombe*. *Gene*, **93**, 265–70.

Viscidi, R. and Shah, K. V. (1992). Immune response to infections with human papillomaviruses. In *Host defence mechanisms*, (ed. T. C. Quinn, J. I. Gallin, and A. S. Fauci), Vol. 8, Raven Press, New York.

Zhou, J., Doorbar, J., Sun, X.Y, Crawford, L. V., McLean, C. S., and Frazer, I. H. (1991). Identification of the nuclear localization signal of human papillomavirus type 16 L1 protein. *Virology*, **185**, 625–32.

8 The search for cell-mediated immunity to HPV: Prospects for vaccine design

HANS J. STAUSS and PETER C. L. BEVERLEY

8.1 What is cell-mediated immunity?

Immune responses may be classified as innate or adaptive, humoral or cellular. Innate responses do not depend on prior exposure for their full effect and are not altered on re-exposure to the same micro-organism. These responses are mediated by non-specific effector mechanisms and cells, such as complement, neutrophils, monocytes, macrophages, dendritic cells, and natural killer (NK) cells. In contrast adaptive responses are antigen specific, often slow and weak on first exposure (primary response), but rapid and effective on re-exposure (secondary or memory response). Adaptive humoral responses depend on antibody secreted by bone-marrow-derived (B) lymphocytes, while most of the cell types involved in innate cellular immunity also take part in adaptive cell-mediated responses. However, the hallmark of adaptive cellular responses is the involvement of antigen-specific thymus-derived (T) lymphocytes.

There is considerable overlap and interplay between innate and adaptive, humoral and cellular responses. Thus for example antibody produced in an adaptive response promotes the phagocytosis of micro-organisms by neutrophils and macrophages of the innate immune system. Antigen presentation by macrophages and dendritic cells in turn activates T cells. Perhaps most importantly, cytokines produced by T cells have a profound effect on the maturation and effector function of almost all non-specific effectors as well as on B lymphocyte production of antibody (helper activity). For this reason this chapter will focus on the role of T lymphocytes in cell-mediated immunity to human papillomaviruses (HPVs) but although the integrated study of all components of cell-mediated immune responses is experimentally not feasible, it is important to acknowledge the limitations of reductionist studies of individual cell types.

Until recently the means by which T cells recognize antigen was not understood but it is now clear that they express heterodimeric T cell receptors (TCR) composed of two chains each with a structure somewhat similar to immunoglobulin light chains. Two types of TCR have been identified. The majority of T cells express $\alpha\beta$ TCR while a minority express a $\gamma\delta$ receptor. While it is clear that $\alpha\beta$ T cells recognize antigen in association with major histocompatibility complex (MHC) class I and II molecules, the nature of the antigen–presenting molecules (restriction elements) for $\gamma\delta$ cells is much less clear.

8.2   Antigen recognition by T lymphocyte

T cells do not recognize intact protein but instead, peptide fragments generated by proteolytic degradation (Townsend *et al.* 1985). These peptides then gain access to cellular compartments were they meet newly synthesized MHC class I or class II molecules, bind to them, and are transported to the cell surface where they are recognized by T lymphocytes as peptide/ MHC complexes. The intracellular compartments for peptide loading of class I and class II molecules are distinct (Fig. 8.1). Peptides in the endoplasmic reticulum (ER) bind class I molecules and stabilize their conformation, which is essential for transport to the golgi compartment and thence to the cell surface. In contrast, class II molecules are prevented from peptide binding in the ER because of their association with invariant chain which is thought to block the peptide binding site. In addition to this blocking function, invariant chain also directs traffic of class II molecules to the endosomal compartment where it is proteolytically cleaved and dissociates from the MHC molecules, allowing them to bind peptides.

It is worth noting that the peptide composition of the endosomal compartment is distinct from that of the ER, which accordingly results in the binding of different sets of peptides by the two classes of MHC molecules. The endosomal compartment contains mostly peptides generated by fragmentation of endocytosed proteins while the ER contains mostly peptides which are generated in the cytosol and transported into the ER. Most cytosolic proteins are synthesized inside the cell while the majority of protein present in endosomes are of extracellular origin. This is why MHC class I molecules preferentially bind peptides derived from proteins produced inside the cell and class II molecules preferentially bind peptides from extracellular proteins. Exceptions to this rule may occur if for example extracellular proteins are delivered into the cytoplasm and thus gain access to the class I presentation pathway.

The two classes of MHC molecules interact with two distinct populations of T cells. Peptides presented by class I stimulate T cells, which express the CD8 accessory molecule. These cells on activation become cytotoxic effector cells (CTL), whose main function is combat intracellular parasites. MHC class II presented peptides are recognized by CD4 expressing lymphocytes, which mediate helper function by secreting immune

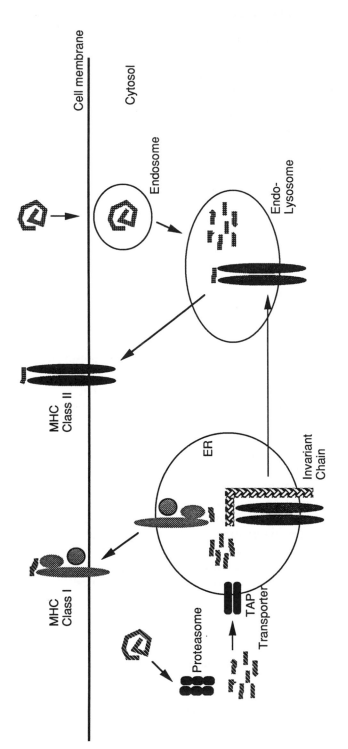

Fig. 8.1 Antigen processing for presentation by MHC class I and II molecules.

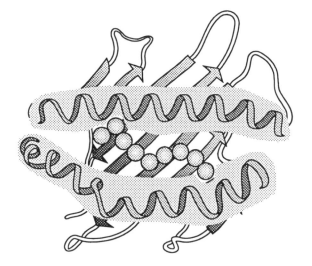

Fig. 8.2 Schematic view of a peptide/MHC complex. The peptide is 9 amino acids long and positions two and nine represent anchor residues which bind to pockets present in the MHC groove. The MHC groove is formed by 8 antiparallel β-sheets topped by two α-helices.

modulating cytokines and are most important in dealing with extracellualr micro-organisms.

The mechanics of peptide/MHC interaction have been worked out very well in the recent past. Two experimental breakthroughs account for this, namely the revelation of the structure of MHC molecules by crystallography (Bjorkman *et al*. 1987) and the direct biochemical analysis of MHC bound peptides (van Bleek and Nathenson 1991, Falk *et al*. 1991). The structure of MHC class I showed that these molecules fold in such a way that the two N-terminal immunoglobulin-like domains form two α-helices which rest on a platform of antiparallel sheets to create a groove in which antigenic peptide fragments are bound (Fig. 8.2). The amino acids lining this peptide binding groove are polymorphic, so that different class I alleles might be expected to bind distinct sets of peptides (Falk *et al*. 1991). Furthermore, the length of the groove provides sufficient space for binding of approximately 9 amino acid long peptides provided they are extended and do not bind in a folded or helical conformation. The features of the peptide binding groove were nicely complemented by direct analysis of MHC bound peptides. It was found that the majority of peptides bound to human and murine class I molecules were 9 amino acids long, except for the murine K^b and K^k molecules which apparently prefer 8mer peptides. Also, distinct peptide pools were isolated from different class I molecules and it was possible to identify allele specific binding motifs. While there may be considerable variation in amino acids at most positions in the 8 or 9 mer peptides bound to a single class I allele, there is much less variation in one or two residues. These have been termed 'anchor residues' and appear to play an important role in peptide binding. Structural analysis shows that the side chains of anchor residues are frequently inserted into pockets in the floor of the antigen binding groove forming stable hydrophobic or hydrogen bond interactions with MHC residues forming the pockets. The position and size of the pockets and thus of the anchor residues varies for different class I alleles.

The crystal structure of the human MHC class II molecule HLA-DR1 has now been resolved. The data show that the folded class II α and β chains form a structure that is highly reminiscent of class I molecules. However, while the class I peptide binding groove is closed at both ends this is not the case for the class II groove. Open ends may allow the amino and carboxyl termini of peptides to extend beyond the binding groove. Analysis of class II bound peptides revealed that they were indeed heterogeneous in size, ranging from 12 to 23 amino acids. Again, specific binding motifs could be identified which apparently mediate the interaction of the peptide core with the class II binding groove. Current evidence suggests that several alleles may bind peptides with similar anchor residues, perhaps providing an explanation for the finding that class II restricted responses often exhibit promiscuous restriction (in other words a given peptide may be presented by several class II alleles).

The practical implication of peptide binding motifs is that they may be used to screen proteins for epitopes that have a high probability of being able to bind to specific MHC class I or class II molecules. Such epitopes are predicted to be immunologically relevant since they might be recognized by T lymphocytes.

8.3   Immune stimulation versus unresponsiveness

The immunological consequences of *in vivo* antigen exposure are critically dependent upon the route and dose of antigen administration. For example, antigen delivery via the oral route or by intravenous injection is often associated with immunological unresponsiveness, while intradermal, subcutaneous, and intramuscular antigen injections often cause immune stimulation. Similarly, high and low antigen doses were classically used to induce unresponsiveness, while intermediate doses lead to immune stimulation. The details of *in vivo* mechanisms governing the outcome of immune responses are not well understood, although the nature of antigen-presenting cells is likely to play a key role. Only specialized immune stimulatory cells are capable of activating antigen-specific T cell responses efficiently, while

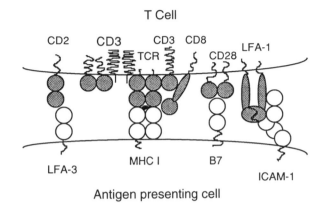

Fig. 8.3 Schematic representation of contact between a T cell and another cell presenting antigen via MHC class 1. Several ligand–receptor pairs are shown. CD3 is a complex of five distinct polypeptide chains with no known ligand but is essential for signal transduction through the T cell receptor. Circles indicate immunoglobulin superfamily domains. Most of these molecules are known to transduce signals across the T cell membrane, indicating the possibilities for subtle regulation of T cell activation or inactivation.

antigen display by non-stimulatory cells fails to activate naive T lymphocytes and can, under experimental *in vitro* conditions, induce unresponsiveness. At present the most likely explanation for failure of many cell types to activate is that although they can present antigen to the TCR they are unable to provide necessary co-stimulatory signals. The exact nature of these essential co-stimuli remains a subject of investigation, but interaction of the T cell surface molecule CD28 with its counter receptor B7 is important, as are several other T cell-antigen presenting cell (APC) interactions (Linsley *et al.* 1990) (Fig. 8.3). Dendritic cells and macrophages are examples of stimulatory cells while fibroblasts, epithelial and neuronal cells are usually non-stimulatory. In the context of HPV immune responses it is worth noting that human keratinocytes have been shown to be poor APCs (Bal *et al.* 1990).

It is possible that different routes and doses of antigen delivery lead to distinct pattern of antigen presentation by stimulatory or non-stimulatory cells, which in turn may determine immune responsiveness. These considerations have practical implications for the administration of vaccines aiming at efficiently inducing immunity. Vaccine design also needs to consider the role of individual cell populations in the induction of immune responses since it might be beneficial to stimulate selectively key regulatory cells. For example, CD4[+] T helper (Th) cells play a central role in the initiation of antigen-specific responses by B lymphocytes and by cytotoxic

T lymphocytes. In fact, at the initiation of immune responses the cytokine profile produced by Th cells will either preferentially stimulate B cells for antibody production or CTL precursors to develop cytotoxic activity. The cytokines IL4 and IL10 are known to stimulate preferentially the former, while IL2 and γIFN efficiently activate the latter. Th cells producing IL2 and γIFN are also the cells which mediate delayed type hypersensitivity (DTH) responses, typified by the skin reaction to mycobacterial antigens. DTH responses contain relatively few antigen-specific T cells and many non-specific effectors. Macrophage activation by γIFN is a prominent feature.

The parameters determining the patterns of Th-produced cytokines are currently unclear, although such knowledge would be extremely useful for controlled immune manipulation. Present evidence suggests that naive Th precursors are not precommitted but that cytokine production is determined by the nature and dose of the antigen and probably by the type of antigen-presenting cells. Operationally, activated effector Th cells which produce IL2 and γIFN have been termed Th1, while secretion of IL4 and IL10 defines Th2 cells (Sher *et al.* 1992). The implications of this dichotomy are that vaccines aiming for the induction of neutralizing antibodies should stimulate Th2 cells, while vaccines for induction of DTH or protective CTL immunity should stimulate Th1 responses. Unfortunately, to date these are theoretical considerations and practical application will depend upon more knowledge of the stimulation requirements of these Th populations. It will also be important to know which responses are important in the control of HPV in humans (see Chapter 10).

8.4   Natural versus induced tumour immunity

In the post-war years Burnett and Thomas restated the theory of immune surveillance, first formulated at the turn of the century. The essence of the hypothesis is that constant monitoring by the immune system allows recognition of transformed cells expressing novel, transformation-associated antigens, leading to immune stimulation and elimination of the altered cells. Thus, the frequency of overt malignancy is low not because of low transformation frequency but because of infrequent escape of transformed cells from immune destruction. Evidence in support of the theory comes from long-term follow-up of immune-suppressed renal transplant patients who show an increased cancer incidence (Sheil 1984). However, occurrence of certain cancers is dramatically increased in these studies while the incidence of others is only marginally increased. A trivial explanation for this could be that the immunosuppressive drugs increase mutation rates in only these tissues showing big increases in cancer incidence. However, the observation that viruses have been implicated in many of the tumours showing increased frequency suggests an immunological explanation. This is that immune surveillance operates against oncogenic viruses, not against transformed cells *per se*. Since warts and carcinoma of the skin and cervix all show an increase in immunosuppressed individuals, this suggests that surveillance operates against HPVs among other viruses.

Despite the doubtful concept of natural immune surveillance, there is little doubt that actively induced immunity can provide tumour protection. Active induction of tumour immunity is dependent on at least two prerequisites; firstly, the existence of antigens that distinguish tumour and normal cells and secondly, the ability of immune effector cells to recognize such antigens. The search for tumour antigens initially focused on the isolation of tumour-specific monoclonal antibodies. The attractive feature of antibodies is that they can be coupled to toxins or radionuclides and thus deliver lethal agents to tumours. However, available monoclonal antibodies are not strictly tumour-specific since they frequently recognize antigens abnormally highly expressed in tumours but also found in some normal tissues. More recently CTL have been used as tools to identify tumour antigens. This approach is particularly exciting since it allows identification of intracellular proteins which are not expressed on the cell surface and therefore not accessible for recognition by antibodies. This is because of the mechanism of intracellular protein breakdown and surface presentation of peptides by MHC class I molecules. It is known that this allows CTL recognition of cytosolic, nuclear, and even mitochondrial proteins, suggesting that there is no hiding place inside cells to escape CTL recognition.

This recognition mechanism allows the immune system to screen tumour cells for intracellular proteins that are distinct from those found in normal cells and to mount a tumour-specific attack. The products of mutated oncogenes and the proteins encoded by transforming viruses are not found in normal cells and provide promising targets for strictly tumour-specific CTL responses. To date, many studies have demonstrated the existence of CTL which can specifically destroy tumour cells, but the target peptides recognized have remained elusive in most cases. One such target peptide, however, was identified in cells of a melanoma patient and it was found to be a 9 amino acid long epitope presented to CTL by HLA-A1 molecules. Surprisingly, this peptide was not derived from a mutated protein but rather from a self protein that was expressed at a high level in melanomas and among normal tissues showed low level expression only in testis (van der Bruggen and Van den Eynde 1992).

In a murine tumour model CTL have been shown to recognize both gene products showing point mutations and over-expressed normal molecules. The knowledge that most tumours show a variety of genetic alterations has also prompted a more directed search for CTL responses to gene products known to be altered in tumours. Promising murine experiments have indicated the potential for immune targeting of altered self proteins by demonstrating CTL which specifically recognize peptides derived from mutant Ras protein (Skipper and Stauss 1993).

CTL are not the only cell type playing an important role in tumour immunity. CD4$^+$ T lymphocytes can sometimes mediate tumour protection and are probably involved in the initiation of most anti-tumour responses where the protective effectors are CD8$^+$ CTL. For example, in murine models where tumour immunity is solely mediated by CD8$^+$ CTL, the initiation of this immunity is often severely compromised in the absence of CD4$^+$ Th cells. Other cell types that have been shown in murine tumour models to have tumour-protective effects are eosinophils, macrophages, and natural killer cells. An important difference in the immunity mediated by these effectors and that by CTL and Th cells is that only the latter develop immunologic memory and can be swiftly reactivated. Nevertheless natural killer cells can be very efficient in providing short-term tumour protection. Although the mechanisms of NK recognition are not fully worked out yet, some fascinating insights have started to emerge (Moretta *et al.* 1992). It has been known for some time that they attack MHC negative cells more efficiently than class I expressing cells. More recently it has been clearly demonstrated that lack of single class I molecules can lead to NK mediated cell lysis even when other class I alleles are expressed normally. Thus, NK cells can potentially attack cancer cells that have lost expression of all or individual MHC class I alleles as is frequently observed in cervical cancers. NK cells probably are not stimulated by absent class I molecules but rather by surface proteins which are exposed when MHC molecules are missing.

Histologic analysis of tumour material frequently demonstrates infiltration of granulocytes, macrophages, and lymphocytes. Attempts to correlate cell types and numbers in tumour infiltrates with the immune status and the prognosis of the disease are questionable. For example, experiments in mice have demonstrated that genetically manipulated tumours expressing IL2, IL4, TNF, γIFN, or GM-CSF are more immunogenic than unmanipulated cells and induce tumour protection (Pardoll 1992). Histologic studies showed that manipulated tumours growing *in vivo* were infiltrated mostly by neutrophils, eosinophils, and macrophages, while T lymphocytes were either absent or very low in numbers. Nevertheless, in all cases, the long-term tumour protection was found to be mediated by CD8$^+$ CTL. It is therefore possible that the tumour tissue is not the site where initiation of long-term immunity occurs, but that infiltrating cells transfer antigen to local lymph nodes for stimulation of T lymphocyte immunity.

8.5 Are there immunogenic CTL epitopes in the E6 and E7 proteins of HPV16?

Transformed cells from patients with HPV 16 associated cervical cancer consistently express the E6 and E7 viral proteins and they appear to be required to maintain the transformed phenotype. This renders them excellent targets for CTL-based immunotherapy, provided that these proteins gain access to the MHC class I presentation pathway and provide immune stimulating peptide epitopes.

Initial experiments designed to investigate whether E6 and E7 are immunogenic have largely been carried out in rodents. Several groups have used similar strategies in which HPV genes products are transfected into rodent cells providing a model for tumour challenge experiments. A variety of immunization strategies have been employed to show that mice and rats can make an immune response to HPV-encoded proteins which is capable of protecting against tumour challenge (Meneguzzi *et al*. 1991). Perhaps most impressive is the protective immunity against an E7-containing murine melanoma cell which can be demonstrated when mice are immunized with the same cell co-transfected with the B7 molecule (the counter receptor for CD28) (Chen *et al*. 1992). Protection in this model is associated with development of a $CD8^+$ CTL response although the exact specificity of this was not determined. Indeed, it is notable that so far no precise epitope mapping of determinants in E6 or E7 has been published, although the fact that protection against challenge with an E7 transfectant can be achieved with a synthetic peptide of the E7 sequence 49–57 (Kast and Melief, personal communication) implies that this may contain a CTL target as well as a known helper epitope (Tindle *et al*. 1991). In our own experiments the E6 and E7 proteins were found to be weakly immunogenic, making it difficult to demonstrate specific CTL responses. For example, mice immunized with E7-transfected cells did not generate detectable CTL responses, which were only seen when mice were immunized with recombinant vaccinia virus expressing E7. This suggests that anti-E7 CTL in HPV 16 positive cancer patients may be difficult to detect. Analysis of the E6- and E7-derived peptides recognized by murine H-2[b] CTL generated against the corresponding proteins also revealed the limitations of predictive peptide motifs. A motif positive peptide of E6 which showed strong MHC class I binding when tested in binding assays was not recognized by anti-E6 CTL, which instead recognized a motif negative peptide that showed only weak class I binding. Lack of response to the motif positive peptide was not due to a 'hole' in the TCR repertoire because the synthetic peptide efficiently stimulated CTL. These peptide-induced CTL were, however, unable to recognize E6 expressing cells, indicating that natural protein processing does not produce this predicted peptide epitope. A similar observation was made with anti-E7 CTL, which recognized a peptide not predicted by motifs instead of a motif-positive epitope. These findings are important for epitope searches in humans, which clearly cannot rely exclusively on the use of synthetic peptides containing motif sequences.

Successful isolation of HPV-specific human CTL depend upon factors that are experimentally controllable but also upon a number of unknown parameters. For example, the *in vivo* immunogenicity of HPV proteins in infected patients is unknown, and murine work suggests that E7 protein is a poor T cell stimulator while E6 appears to be more efficient. This raises the possibility that HPV proteins other than E6 and E7 are more immunogenic in humans and may dominate T cell responses. Furthermore, it is currently unknown which effector cells will be efficient *in vivo* in eliminating HPV-expressing cells. Although CD8$^+$ CTL are efficient in many tumour systems, CD4$^+$ Th cells can potentially mediate tumour protection due to their ability to recruit and activate macrophages, natural killer cells, and other leukocytes. Another intriguing question is, at what stage of HPV infection is T cell immunity stimulated? Serologic studies have suggested that levels of HPV-specific antibodies correlate with the severity of HPV-associated disease (see Chapter 7). It would appear that the responses measured in these studies were a consequence of large tumour burden rather than immunity initiated at early disease stages. Obviously, only such early occurring responses may counteract disease progression and consequently improve patients' prognosis.

Analysis of T lymphocyte immunity to HPV infection serves two major goals. A primary concern is whether is it possible to identify any immunogenic epitopes in HPV proteins that are recognized by human T cells, which would allow an approach to secondary questions such as, do these epitopes stimulate T cells in patients and at what stage of disease, and can these epitopes be used to induce specific immunity in patients? To tackle the first question lymphocytes from surgically removed tumours, draining lymph nodes, or peripheral blood can be stimulated *in vitro* with autologous APCs expressing HPV proteins. Protein expression can be achieved by infecting APCs with recombinant vaccinia or adenovirus constructs expressing HPV proteins. Using naturally processed protein for T cell stimulation overcomes a bias that is introduced when using synthetic peptides, which are selected based on MHC binding motifs or binding assays. Recombinant viruses are suitable for channelling HPV proteins into the MHC class I presentation pathway for recognition by CTL, while recombinant protein produced in bacterial or eukaryotic expression systems is suitable for class II presentation and stimulation of Th cells. Once protein-specific CTL or Th are isolated epitope mapping can be achieved rapidly using synthetic peptides. Initial studies using this approach have shown that it is feasible to identify at least MHC class II presented epitopes (Altmann *et al.* 1992). An alternative is to isolate natural peptides from MHC molecules of protein expressing cells. This latter approach is particularly useful because it allows detection of multiple T cell epitopes which might go unnoticed when limited sets of synthetic peptides are used for screening.

Passing the hurdle of identifying immunogenic epitopes presented by HLA class I and class II molecules will allow more specific analysis of immune status in patients. Synthetic peptides corresponding to identified epitopes can be used to monitor all patients expressing appropriate HLA molecules to evaluate whether or not they harbour epitope-specific T lymphocytes. It will become practical to monitor large numbers of patients to correlate presence or absence of T cell immunity with stage and severity of disease. Identification of epitopes will obviously affect vaccine design.

8.6 What vaccine and when?

Immunological intervention in papillomavirus-related disease can be envisaged at several different stages. Prevention of infection by prophylactic vaccination is appealing but presents several difficulties. It seems likely that such a vaccine would need to induce neutralizing antibody but as yet there is no assay for virus neutralization and although the capsid proteins (L1 and L2) appear to be the obvious targets, the virus receptor for cells has not been defined. In addition, since it is likely that the target for neutralization would be epitopes present on native capsid proteins (L1 and L2), candidate vaccines should most likely contain these proteins in a form approximating to native viral particles. Although small quantities of recombinant 'virus-like' empty particles have been produced, scale up would be a formidable task. Further difficulties in the use of such a prophylactic vaccine would be in defining when and to whom to administer it and how to formulate a vaccine intended to induce primarily mucosal immunity.

Alternative vaccine strategies aim to interfere with progression of disease after infection has become established. Since these are aimed at infected or transformed cells their targets need not be antigens expressed in the assembled virus. The early gene products, E6 and E7, which are retained even in transformed cells, are attractive targets but other early genes such as E4 are transcribed in HPV-related lesions (Chapters 5 and 6). Since these are intracellular proteins it is likely that to be effective any vaccine must aim to induce CTL, although a CD4-mediated delayed type hypersensitivity response may also play an important role (Chapters 10 and 11). Intervention can be envisaged at two stages of disease, either for treatment of CIN or overt carcinoma. In the latter case immunotherapy could be viewed as adjuvant treatment to be used following primary debulking surgery. Trials of candidate vaccines to be used in this setting are near to commencement in the UK and elsewhere.

While it is possible to decide on likely candidate antigens for vaccines the choice of formulation of the vaccine is much more difficult. The difficulties of producing native proteins in sufficient quantities and of targeting vaccination to induce appropriate mucosal immunity have already been touched on. For therapeutic vaccines, aimed at inducing a CTL response, the antigen must be targeted to the class I pathway of antigen presentation. Live virus vectors, e.g. vaccinia virus (Moss 1991), do this effectively but the use of vaccinia raises safety issues and if the host has already encountered the unmodified virus, the effectiveness of the response to the recombinant containing the target antigen may be modified. Other virus vectors are under consideration and several bacterial vectors have been proposed, including disabled salmonella and mycobacteria. The efficacy of these in generating CTL remains to be conclusively established. Human cells are also a potential vector for CTL target antigens but have the disadvantage that they need to express the same MHC class I antigens as the host. Although at first sight this appears a major drawback a relatively small panel of transfected cells expressing a few of the most common alleles would cover much of the population.

There remain two other possibilities. The first is the use of synthetic peptides. In mice, immunization with single peptide epitopes has been shown capable of protecting against virus infection and also against challenge with tumour cells containing transfected adenovirus genes as target tumour-associated antigens. In the same model it has been demonstrated that a CTL clone is capable of eradicating an established tumour when passively transferred to the tumour-bearing animal with recombinant interleukin-2 (Greenberg 1991; Melief 1992). Preliminary data suggests that similar protection against challenge with a tumour transfected with HPV E7 can be obtained by immunizing with an E7-derived synthetic peptide (Kast and Melief, personal communication). There is thus no doubt that immunization with synthetic peptides can be effective but in humans this strategy presents the problem that few target epitopes for HPV responses have been defined and different epitopes will be needed for optimal presentation by different MHC alleles.

A possible novel vaccine strategy is the presentation of antigens by direct injection of the genes coding for them. This offers the advantages, also possessed by whole cells, that co-stimulatory molecules can be incorporated into the DNA construct and that antigens are likely to be well presented by the class I pathway. Experience with the methodology is as yet limited but it appears promising (Ulmer *et al.* 1993).

8.7   Conclusions and questions

Whether the aim is development of a prophylactic vaccine or immunotherapy, HPV presents several challenges. Some of these are of a purely technical nature. Thus it is presently impossible to grow large quantities of most HPV types *in vitro* or in animals so that assays depending on the availability of native proteins are made difficult, although advances in recombinant technology promise to overcome this. There are similar problems in assaying CTL responses. The use of recombinant viral vectors, e.g. vaccinia, for *in vitro* boosting or assay has the disadvantage that a response to the vector may make detection of weak HPV-specific responses difficult. Transfectants do not always express high levels of the introduced genes and may be unstable. In principle the exploitation of predictive algorithms and synthetic peptides should circumvent many of these obstacles but in practice the predicted peptides are not always recognized in natural responses. It is partly these technical difficulties which account for the paucity of data on human T cell responses to HPV.

There may, however, be additional reasons for difficulties in detecting human as opposed to mouse responses to HPV gene products. In humans HPV infection is largely confined to cells of stratified squamous epithelium and although this contains specialized antigen-presenting dendritic cells, there is no information on the efficiency of presentation of HPV antigens to the immune system by this route. It is striking that the frequency and magnitude of antibody responses to many HPV antigens increases with severity of HPV-associated disease and our preliminary data suggests that this may be the case for helper T cell responses also. This may imply that the systemic immune response to HPV may be both antigen dose dependent and perhaps also potentiated when there is breakdown of the basement membrane of the epithelium and more ready systemic presentation of antigen. There may also be a local immune response to HPV which is not reflected in readily detectable responses in the blood. A final additional possibility is that HPV, like many other viruses, adopts strategies that minimize immune response to it, e.g. by interfering with antigen presentation, although as yet no such mechanisms have been defined for HPV.

These difficulties suggest that for rational development of either immunotherapy or a prophylactic vaccine we need to know much more about the human immune response to HPV. In particular it will be important to define: (1) the nature of local immune responses to HPV; (2) target epitopes for CTL and helper T cells which can be presented by common HLA alleles; (3) which immune response are effective in protection from infection or therapy of HPV-related diseases (perhaps most easily investigated in genital warts rather than carcinoma of the cervix, see Chapter 11); (4) what formulation of vaccine antigens is most effective in inducing appropriate immune responses?

While these may be difficult questions to answer fully, HPV and carcinoma of the cervix do present the great advantage for tumour immunologists that there are well-defined target tumour associated antigens and in the last few years there has been encouraging progress in understanding T cell and antibody responses to HPV.

References

Altmann, A., Jochmus-Kudielka, I., Rainer, F., Gausepohl, H., Moebius, U., Gissmann, L. *et al.* (1992). Definition of immunogenic determinants of the human papillomavirus type 16 nucleoprotein E7. *European Journal of Cancer*, **28**, 326–33.

Bal, V., McIndoe, A., Denton, G., Hudson, D., Lombardi, G., Lamb, J. *et al.* (1990). Antigen presentation by keratinocytes induces tolerance in human T cells. *European Journal of Immunology*, **20**, 1893–7.

Bjorkman, P. J., Saper, M. A., Samraoui, B., Bennett, W. S., Strominger, J. L., and Wiley, D. C. (1987). The foreign antigen binding site and T cell recognition regions of class I histocompatibility antigens. *Nature*, **329**, 512–18.

Chen, L., Ashe, A., Brady, W. A., Hellstrom, I., Hellstrom, K. E., Ledbetter, J. A., *et al.* (1992). Costimulation of antitumor immunity by the B7 counter-receptor for the T lymphocyte molecules CD28 and CTLA-4. *Cell*, **71**, 1093–102.

Falk, K., Rötzschke, O., Stevanovic, S., Jung, G., and Rammensee, H.-G. (1991). Allele-specific motifs revealed by sequencing of self-peptides eluted from MHC molecules. *Nature*, **351**, 290–6.

Greenberg, P. D. (1991). Adoptive T cell therapy of tumors: mechanisms operative in the recognition and elimination of tumor cells. *Advances in Immunology*, **48**, 281–355.

Linsley, P. S., Clark, E. A., and Ledbeller, J. A. (1990). T-cell antigen CD28 mediates adhesion with B cells by interacting with activation anitigen B7/BB-1. *Proceedings of the National Academy of Sciences (USA)*, **87**, 5031–5.

Melief, C. J. M. (1992). Tumor eradication by adoptive transfer of cytotoxic T lymphocytes. *Advances in Cancer Research*, **58**, 143–75.

Meneguzzi, G., Cerni, C., Kieny, M. P., and Lathe, R. (1991). Immunization against human papillomavirus type 16 tumor cells with recombinant vaccinia viruses expressing E6 and E7. *Virology*, **181**, 62–9.

Moretta, L., Ciccone, E., Moretta, A., Hoglund, P., Ohlen, C., and Karre, K. (1992). Allorecognition by NK cells: nonself or no self? *Immunology Today*, **13**, 300–6.

Moss, B. (1991). Vaccinia virus: a tool for research and vaccine development. *Science-Washington*, **252**, 1662–7.

Pardoll, D. (1992). New strategies for active immunotherapy with genetically engineered tumor cells. *Current Opinion in Immunology*, **4**, 619–23.

Sheil, A. G. R. (1984). Cancer in organ transplant recipients: part of an induced immune deficiency syndome. *British Medical Journal*, **288**, 659–61.

Sher, A., Gazzinelli, R. T., Oswald, I. P., Clerici, M., Kullberg, M., Pearce, E. J., *et al.* (1992). Role of T-cell derived cytokines in the downregulation of immune responses in parasitic and retroviral infection. *Immunological Reviews*, **127**, 183–204.

Skipper, J. and Stauss, H. J. (1993). Identification of two cytotoxic T lymphocyte-recognised epitopes in the Ras protein. *Journal of Experimental Medicine*, **177**, 1493–8.

Tindle, R. W., Fernando, G. J., Sterling, J. C., and Frazer, I. H. (1991). A 'public' T-helper epitope of the E7 transforming protein of human papillomavirus 16 provides cognate help for several E7 B-cell epitopes from cervical cancer-associated human papillomavirus genotypes. *Proceedings of the National Academy of Sciences (USA)*, **88**, 5887–91.

Townsend, A. R., Gotch, F. M., and Davey, J. (1985). Cytotoxic T cells recognize fragments of the influenza nucleoprotein. *Cell*, **42**, 457–67.

Ulmer, J. B., Donnelly, J. J., Parker, S. E., Rhodes, G. H., Felgner, P. L., Dwarki, V. J., Gromkowski, S. H., Deck, R. R., Dewitt, C. M., and Friedman, A. (1993). Heterologous protection against influenza by injection of DNA encoding a viral protein. *Science*, **259**, 1745–9.

van Bleek, G. and Nathenson, S. (1991). The structure of the antigen-binding groove of major histocompatibility complex class I molecules determines specific selection of self-peptides. *Proceedings of the National Academy of Sciences (USA)*, **88**, 11032–6.

van der Bruggen, P. and Van den Eynde, B. (1992). Molecular definition of tumor antigens recognised by T lymphocytes. *Current Opinion in Immunology*, **4**, 608–12.

9 MHC expression in the natural history of cervical cancer

PETER L. STERN and MARGARET DUGGAN-KEEN

9.1 Introduction

An active role of the immune system in preventing the development of HPV-associated malignancies is supported by evidence that immuno-compromised individuals such as allograft recipients, cancer and AIDS patients exhibit an increased incidence of HPV-associated lesions (Schneider and Koutsky 1992). Immunological intervention might therefore be a useful approach to the control and prevention of cervical neoplasia.

It is likely that the T cell mediated arm of the immune response would be of primary importance in any surveillance of tumour cells. The most likely viral target antigens would be derived from the HPV16/18 E6 and E7 transforming genes which are frequently retained and expressed in cervical carcinomas (see Chapter 5). The recognition of foreign peptide antigens by T cells is restricted by the polymorphic products of the major histocompatibility complex (MHC) class I and class II products. The HLA-A, -B, and -C loci encode the MHC class I polymorphic 45kD heavy chains which associate with an invariant 12kD β2-microglobulin chain. They are expressed by most somatic cells and present antigens synthesized endogenously (e.g viral products) as processed peptides to CD8 cytotoxic T cells (Bjorkman *et al.* 1987; Chapter 8). The HLA- DR, -DP, and -DQ loci encode the MHC class II heterodimeric α (32kD) and β (28kD) chain complexes and are expressed primarily by antigen-presenting cells but also by some epithelia. They can present processed peptides from both exogenous and endogenous antigens to CD4 helper T cells (Neefjes and Ploegh 1992). Both HLA class I and II expression can be up-regulated by various cytokines (Burke *et al.* 1993).

Since MHC molecules play such a central role in presenting potential immunogenic peptides to T cells, altered expression by tumour cells may directly influence immunosurveillance mechanisms. There is extensive information concerning the alteration of HLA expression in many different tumour systems (Garrido and Ruiz-Cabello 1991). Tumours frequently exhibit loss of expression when derived from HLA class I positive mucosa but may also upregulate HLA expression when derived from HLA negative or weakly expressing tissues. Similarly, HLA class II antigen positive tumours can be derived from a negative mucosa. The relationship to prognosis of such changes varies with tumour types and can be favourable, disadvantageous, or of no apparent significance. In view of the association between carcinoma of the cervix and HPV infection, changes in expression of MHC class I or II molecules in the tumours might have important implications for presentation of viral target antigens to the immune system.

This chapter reviews the evidence for alterations in HLA class I and II expression in premalignant and malignant cervical lesions. The possible direct influence of HPV infection/gene expression and other possible mechanisms leading to modulation of HLA in cervical disease are examined. Finally the implications for immunosurveillance of HPV/cervical cancer and prophylactic or therapeutic immunizations are discussed.

9.2 HLA class I and II expression in premalignant and malignant squamous epithelial lesions of the cervix

Figure 9.1 illustrates the disease continuum in cervical cancer and pre-cancer, ranging from CIN through micro-invasion to invasive carcinoma; about 70 per cent of the tumours are squamous and 30 per cent adeno- and adenosquamous carcinomas (Chapter 1). Most tumours are thought to develop from an area of intra-epithelial neoplasia within the transformation zone. This is at the junction of the ectocervical non-keratinizing stratified squamous epithelium and the columnar epithelium lining the endocervical canal. At puberty, the increased concentration of ovarian hormones increases the bulk of the cervix, leading to eversion of the columnar epithelium. Squamous metaplasia, the gradual replacement of the columnar by squamous epithelium through reserve cell proliferation, occurs in response to the relative acidity of the vaginal environment compared to that of the cervical canal. It is in the transformation zone that CIN may arise either by unicellular origin with horizontal spread to replace the normal epithelium or by field transformation.

The expression of MHC products in tumours has been primarily investigated by immunohistochemical methods. Figure 9.1 summarizes work from this laboratory (Connor and Stern 1990; Glew *et al.* 1992a, 1993a; P. Keating, unpublished) from analysis of HLA class I expression with W6/32 monoclonal antibody (mAb) in cryostat and HLA class II expression by mAb CR3/43 in cryostat and paraffin embedded sections of various cervical lesions representing the natural history of squamous carcinoma of the cervix. These reagents recognize monomorphic determinants of the heterodimeric HLA class I or II locus products respectively. The HLA molecules can also be detected using antibodies that recognize chain specific, locus specific, or polymorphic determinants.

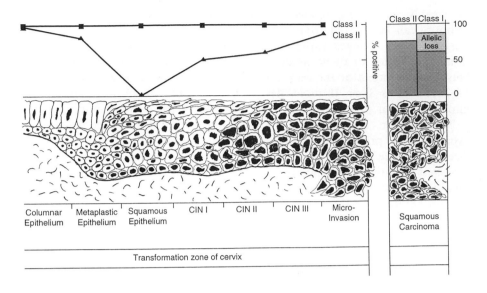

Fig. 9.1 Natural history of HLA expression in cervical lesions. HLA class II expression decreases during the normal maturation process to squamous epithelium in the transformation zone. The proportion of lesions expressing HLA class II correlates with increasing dysplasia. HLA class I expression is apparently unchanged in pre-invasive disease, but is lost in a proportion of carcinomas.

To date 11 per cent (17/155) of the squamous cell carcinomas (SCC) of the cervix have shown a loss of HLA-A,-B, -C and β_2-microglobulin complexed molecules in part or all of the tumour. However, using allele specific mAbs, a further proportion of these biopsies have been shown to exhibit down-regulation of particular allelic products (Connor and Stern 1990). Overall, altered HLA class I expression is probably present in at least 40 per cent of the carcinomas. In another study analysing HLA expression in SCC with paraffin embedded material, using mAb HC10 which recognizes free heavy chains of class I molecules, a greater level of class I down-regulation has been reported (Cromme *et al.* 1993a). However, this might reflect differential allelic expression (HC10 sees mainly HLA-B, -C heavy chains) or lower sensitivity (comparison in frozen sections of HC10 with W6/32, unpublished observations) or since the HC10 determinant is masked by association with β_2-microglobulin, reduced HC10 reactivity might imply increased HLA class I complex expression.

Interpretation of altered HLA class I expression in cervical lesions is less ambiguous with W6/32 in cryostat sections since this reagent should detect all functional HLA class I molecules. It is therefore surprising that virtually all benign and premalignant lesions of cervical epithelia analysed are HLA class I positive; a single exception was a full thickness loss in a grade II CIN (cervical intra-epithelial neoplasm) (Glew *et al.* 1993a). It is possible that this low frequency of HLA class I down-regulation compared to the invasive tumours may reflect the inadequencies of assessing HLA expression by immunohistochemistry. This would be exacerbated by heterogeneity of HLA expression within a lesion and by the likelihood that not all such lesions are progressive. However, it is estimated that some 30 per cent of CIN III (carcinoma *in situ*) lesions will progress to invasive disease if not treated (McIndoe *et al.* 1984). If this were a true indication of progression in cervical malignancy then one might have expected to see more of the specimens examined to show HLA class I loss. It is possible that the latter changes reflect important events that occur at the step that breeches the threshold of invasion and this is supported by data from breast, colon, and lung tumours and their premalignant lesions (Garrido *et al.* 1993).

As can be seen from Fig. 9.1, the HLA class II phenotypes of cervical epithelia change with differentiation and disease. In the transformation zone, reserve cells become apparent at the first stage of squamous metaplasia and the three cases of hyperplasia studied were class II positive as were 80 per cent of cases of immature squamous metaplasia (Glew *et al.* 1993a). It is tempting to speculate that class II molecules are down-regulated during the maturation process to mature squamous epithelium in the transformation zone. The proportions of HLA class II positive specimens of squamous epithelia in cervical lesions exhibiting CIN increases with the severity of the dysplasia.

It appears that local cytokine production is not the sole cause of the epithelial cell class II expression since there is a sharp demarcation of class II expression at the interface of CIN III/normal squamous epithelium in some specimens. Also there is a lack of correspondence of class II expression with heavy sub-epithelial leucocyte infiltration (e.g. in 'chronic active cervicitis') in normal epithelium, CIN, or HPV infection (HPVI) (Glew *et al.* 1993a). In contrast to normal squamous cervical epithelium, the majority (81 per cent, 137/169; Fig. 9.1) of squamous cervical carcinomas express HLA class II antigens in all or a proportion of the tumour cells. Although tumours in the adeno- and adenosquamous carcinoma groups may be glandular in origin (HLA class II positive), approximately the same distribution of class II phenotypes is found as for the SCC (Glew *et al.* 1992a).

9.3 Modulation of HLA expression in relation to HPV DNA in cervical lesions

Squamous carcinomas of the cervix frequently show alterations in the expression of HLA class I and/or class II molecules when compared to the normal epithelium from which they are derived. Are these changes the result of the direct influence of the HPV infections associated with these cancers?

A large proportion of cervical carcinomas contain DNA of HPV type 16 (and 18) but no association between HPV DNA and HLA class I and II changes seen in the cervical carcinomas has been found (Connor and Stern, 1990; Glew *et al.* 1992a). This does not exclude a relationship between HPV gene function and HLA class I or II expression. The study of Cromme *et al.* (1993a) and has established that there is no obligate correlation between transcription of HPV 16 E7 detected by *in situ* hybridization and changes in HLA heavy chain expression in cervical carcinomas.

The pathogenesis of cervical cancer is a multifactorial, multistage process and MHC expression might show a relationship to HPV infection in the evolution of premalignant disease. Indeed, a recent study (Glew *et al.* 1993a) showed that, while high-risk HPV (16, 18, 31, 33) types are not detected in normal or metaplastic epithelia with or without warty changes, there is an increase in the detection in CIN I (27 per cent), CIN II (54 per cent), and CIN III (79 per cent), which parallels the change in HLA class II expression (Fig. 9.1). However, there was no correlation between the groups of cervical lesions exhibiting either no HPV, low or high-risk HPV infections, and the HLA class II phenotypes. This suggests that the latter is not a consequence or a requirement of HPV infection in the cervix. Detection of high-risk HPV DNA in cervical premalignant lesions is also clearly not associated with any change in HLA class I expression.

9.4   Strategies for HLA modulation in tumours

The above studies only correlate the presence of viral DNA (RNA) with MHC expression whereas the viral protein expression may be the critical element. The latter may directly or indirectly lead to MHC class I and/or II changes in cervical tumours. All or some of the following mechanisms may contribute to alterations in MHC expression in cervical cancer.

9.4.1   HLA class I

Some adenoviruses are able to influence the expression of MHC class I at the transcriptional level by the action of the early region gene product E1A (Schrier *et al.* 1983). This does not appear to be a mechanism utilized by papillomaviruses even though E7 and E1A show strong sequence similarity. While HPV E6 and E7 transforming functions involve interaction with cellular tumour suppressors p53 and Rb respectively, there are no known consequences of the latter for MHC expression. Regulation of

HLA class I expression may result from the subsequent influence on other cellular oncogene products (see Chapter 5).

In melanomas, for example, upregulation of c-myc, which encodes a leucine zipper type transcription factor, correlates with reduced HLA-B locus expression (Versteeg *et al.* 1989). Sequencing of upstream regulatory regions of HLA reveal differences between alleles and between loci (Schmidt *et al.* 1990). Perhaps there is an altered transcriptional regulatory programme with a differential effect on HLA-B expression. It is possibly relevant that in invasive genital cancers, HPV genomes are preferentially integrated near myc genes (Couturier *et al.* 1991). HPV influenced upregulation of c-myc expression might mediate the HLA down-regulation in a proportion of cervical carcinomas. However, c-myc overexpression does not always correlate directly with class I loss at either the transcriptional or protein level (Cromme *et al.* 1993b).

Is it possible that post-transcriptional mechanisms account for the many cases of HLA class I down-regulation seen in cervical cancer? Indeed the study of Cromme *et al.* (1993) indicated that modulation of HLA expression is not transcriptionally controlled in cervical carcinomas. Figure 9.2 (see also Fig. 8.1) shows the major events leading to the surface display of class I heavy chain-peptide-β_2m complexes (Monaco 1992). The translated heavy chains are translocated to the lumen of the endoplasmic reticulum, core glycosylated, and bind allele-compatible peptides (usually 9mers). These peptides are generated from endogenously synthesized proteins (e.g. virus) in the cytoplasm, possibly by components of the proteosome coded in the MHC and transported to the lumen of the ER via a specific ABC type transporter associated with antigen processing. This peptide transporter is composed of TAP 1/2 subunits encoded by genes in the MHC (Kelly *et al.* 1992). When peptides bind to specific HLA heavy chains there are conformational changes which are stabilized by the binding of β_2m molecules (Townsend *et al.* 1990). On reaching the Golgi the high mannose sugars of the heavy chain are processed and complex sugars added. This step allows the transport of the tri-molecular complex to the cell surface.

A precedent for viral modulation of functional MHC expression by inhibition of the transport of peptide-loaded MHC complex class I molecules into the medial-Golgi compartment has been described recently (De Val *et al.* 1992). The effect of early cytomegalovirus (CMV) gene expression is to inhibit further glycosylation of MHC class I molecules so preventing the transport of these molecules through the Golgi compartment thus interfering with the natural pathway for the processing and presentation of CMV-derived antigenic peptides. Adenovirus uses a related strategy for effects on intracellular transport of MHC class I molecules. A retention signal is contained within the six COOH-terminal amino acids of the E3/19K protein of adenovirus 2 and mediates the ER/*cis*-Golgi retention of complexes betwen E3/19K and MHC class I molecules; interestingly alleles

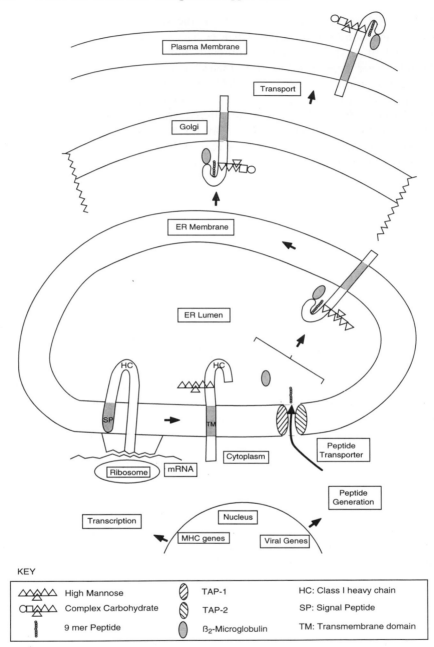

Fig. 9.2 Major events leading to the surface expression of HLA class I molecules. Peptides generated from endogenously synthesized proteins (eg. virus) are transported to the lumen of the ER, via the TAP1/TAP2 transporter. Binding of

Fig. 9.2   (*continued*)

allele-specific peptide to class I heavy chain together with β_2-microglobulin forms a stable tri-molecular complex which is processed in the Golgi to the mature glycosylated form and then transported to the cell surface.

vary in susceptibility to E3/19K (Cox *et al.* 1991). Our studies of HPV 16 transfected keratinocytes (Bartholomew *et al.* 1994) have shown an increased free heavy chain expression detected by HC10 mAb which could be consistent with an altered ability of some heavy chain molecules to associate with β_2-microglobulin (Neefjes and Ploegh 1988). To locate any possible effect on post-translational modification of HLA class I molecules in the HPV 16 transfected keratinocytes, the susceptibility of MHC molecules to Endo-H digestion was determined. This enzyme preferentially cleaves immature N-linked oligosaccharides characteristic of glycoproteins that have not reached the medial-Golgi compartment. However, it appears that HPV 16 does not interfere in the production of mature glycosylated class I molecules in these keratinocytes.

Any disturbance of heavy chain-peptide interactions and their subsequent stabilization by β_2-microglobulin would have direct consequences for potential immune recognition of tumour target antigens. Surface expression of HLA class I molecules is known to be deficient in cell lines that have defective TAP1 or TAP2 gene products (Kelly *et al.* 1992; Townsend *et al.* 1990). This results from the lack of appropriate peptides in the ER lumen which could interact with the specific polymorphic class I molecules leading to their surface expression. It is possible that HPV gene expression could interfere with the TAP gene function, leading to down-regulation of class I expression. This might manifest itself at an allelic level since there is clearly allelic variation in efficiency of assembly of HLA class I products (Neefjes and Ploegh 1988). Some small cell carcinomas of the lung have functional down-regulation of TAP products, producing MHC class I reduction and lack of peptide presentation (Restifo *et al.* 1993). Recent studies have shown a strong correlation between TAP-1 gene expression and down-regulation of HLA class I products in cervical cancer (Cromme *et al.* 1994).

Such mechanisms are unlikely to account for all the MHC class I down-regulation. At least a proportion of HLA negative tumours result from the absence of β_2-microglobulin expression (Garrido and Ruiz-Cabello 1991). Surprisingly in our study (Connor and Stern 1990) β_2-microglobulin was often accompanied by the absence of HLA heavy chains. These observations suggest that the regulation of expression of several gene products associated with MHC expression must be altered in cervical cancer. In development it has been shown that MHC class I and β_2-microglobulin expression is primarily regulated at the transcriptional level (Drezen *et al.* 1993). The diversity of transcription factors and their genetic response elements which are shared by many of the different MHC components (e.g. interferon regulated expression of class I, II, TAP, etc.) might account for the complex phenotypes observed.

It is possible that the down-regulation of HLA class I may be the result of immunoselective events, advantageous to the evolution of an invasive cancer. If this were true then it follows that those HLA allelic products capable of presenting target peptides of, for example, HPV 16 E6/E7 would be preferentially lost. This phenotype could be produced as a result of interference at any level in the regulation of expression of HLA. Thus the tumours with an HLA class I down-regulated phenotype, as assessed by immunohistochemistry, could be very heterogeneous in their defects.

9.4.2   HLA class II

What accounts for the upregulation of HLA class II expression in squamous epithelia of cervical premalignant and malignant lesions? It is not possible to exclude that HPV gene function might influence this HLA class II expression directly. A more likely possibility is that the expression of HLA class II by the majority of SCC is coincidental to HPV infection in the transformation zone. Since most SCC are thought to develop from the transformation zone which undergoes the physiological process of squamous metaplasia during which class II expression is presumably regulated, it is possible that the distribution of tumour class II phenotypes is the result of selection and fixation at the stage at which 'transformation' takes place. The precise origin of the reserve cells remains unknown but it is possible that they represent the target cell type for origin of premalignant lesions of the cervix. Adenocarcinoma *in situ* arises in the columnar cells of the endocervix and is thought to be the precursor lesion of at least a proportion of adenocarcinomas. The fact that the patterns of class II expression are similar for squamous and adeno/adenosquamous tumours could be the result of common features in the origins and/or natural history of these different tumour pathological types.

The biological function and clinical implications of MHC class II expression by the squamous epithelium in cervical disease is unknown. The HLA class II expression observed in cervical lesions is likely to be constitutive, but the fact that HLA class II molecules can be expressed by normal keratinocytes in response to cytokines is consistent with a functional role in antigen presentation (Nickoloff *et al.* 1993). Optimal activation of specific T cells requires that in addition to MHC presentation of peptide antigen other accessory molecule interactions must occur between the antigen-presenting cell and the T cell (see also Chapter 8). For example, ICAM-1 promotes adhesion in immunological interactions by acting as the ligand for the integrin molecule LFA-1, expressed on T lymphocytes. LFA-1 is required for a wide range of leucocyte functions including T cell-mediated killing, T-helper, and B-lymphocyte responses. LFA-3 acts as the ligand for the T cell specific LFA-2 (CD2) antigen. Both the LFA-1/target ICAM-1 pathway and the LFA-2/target LFA-3 pathways are required for optimal effector/target conjugation—in this case effective T-helper or cytotoxic T-cell/tumour cell conjugation (Springer 1990). LFA-3 is expressed by normal squamous epithelium whereas ICAM-1 is upregulated in neoplastic cervical squamous epithelium. The tumour areas expressing class II determinants usually label positively for the cellular adhesion molecule ICAM-1 and class II-associated invariant chain (Ii). The role of invariant chain is believed to control the intracellular transport of class II MHC molecules from the endoplasmic reticulum, through the Golgi apparatus into an endosomal compartment where it is suggested class II molecules meet endocytosed exogenous antigens (Neefjes and Ploegh 1992). Here, in the low pH, Ii is released and this allows the peptides to interact with the α and β chain complex of the class II molecules; these complexes are subsequently transported to the cell surface. It seems that this display of immunoregulatory molecules by the neoplastic cervical epithelium could function in antigen presentation to infiltrating T cells.

Indeed, it has been shown that keratinocytes can function as accessory cells in response to superantigens (Nickoloff *et al.* 1993). Such antigen presentation may result in immunofacilitation by class II restricted T-helper/ inducer lymphocytes, for example leading to specific antibody responses. Thus one possibility would be that areas of CIN or HPVI expressing HLA class II molecules would be more likely to regress than their class II negative counterparts.

However, in some circumstances antigen presentation by keratinocytes induces tolerance in human T cells (Bal *et al.* 1990). Such observations may reflect the requirement for additional co-stimulatory signals for T-cell activation provided by the interaction of the B7 ligand expressed by antigen-presenting cells and CD28 receptors on T cells (Harding *et al.* 1992). In the absence of these signals, a state of anergy is induced in the specific T cells. It is not yet clear whether keratinocytes can express functional B7 molecules (Nickoloff *et al.* 1993) so it is possible that inadequacy in co-stimulatory signals modulates immunity to HPV in cervical disease. Such immunosuppressive effects would exacerbate the already impaired afferent arm of the immune system resulting from the reduced epithelial Langerhans' cells (professional antigen-presenting cells) present in CIN (Hughes *et al.* 1988). Thus HLA class II positive lesions might be more likely to persist or progress than their negative counterparts. Follow up studies may give an indication of any clinical implications but the complexity of positive and negative MHC related influences may obscure any clear indication.

9.5   HLA polymorphism

Associations between certain HLA antigens and many diseases have been established although only weakly with several different cancers. The MHC restriction of T cell recognition of antigen probably functions at the molecular level by the selection of short peptide sequences for binding to HLA and this is influenced by the polymorphic sites (Bjorkman *et al.* 1987; Rudensky *et al.* 1991). Since different alleles will present different peptides to the immune system, the loss (or up-regulation) of individual alleles may influence the natural history of HPV infection and subsequent development of cervical malignancy. If this is the case, it would be reflected in a different spectrum of HLA antigen frequencies in patients with cervical disease compared to the normal population. A recent article (Wank and Thomssen 1991) has claimed the association of HLA-DQ3 and HLA-DR5, the latter possibly as a result of linkage disequilibrium, with increased risk of squamous carcinoma of the cervix. A significant decrease in the frequency of HLA-DR6 was also noted. The association with HLA-DQ3 has been confirmed in a study from Norway with a smaller relative risk (Helland *et al.* 1992). In our studies (Glew *et al.* 1992a, 1993b), there were no statistically significant associations of any HLA-A, -B, -Cw, DR, or -DQ serologically defined antigen with cervical cancer. Specifically, there was no increase in frequency of HLA-DQ3 or decrease in frequency of HLA-DR6 in our patient group, although the frequency of these antigens in control populations in the Manchester and German studies were similar. Possible explanations of the differences between the German and our similar sized studies may lie in an unintentional selection of either patient or control groups. Alternatively, different viral factors may be involved in the development of cervical cancers in Britain as compared to southern Germany. It is also possible that there is microheterogeneity of HLA-DQ molecules in the two populations which might influence susceptibility but molecular typing rather than serology does not explain the differences (Glew *et al.* 1993b; Wank *et al.* 1992). It is therefore unclear whether HLA-DQ3 is truly a susceptibility gene for cervical cancer.

A further analysis of our squamous carcinoma patient HLA data with various tumour cell phenotypes has indicated a trend for certain HLA antigens to associate with subgroups of patients defined by MHC tumour phenotype (HLA class I or II negative or homogeneously/heterogeneously positive). The study size is the limiting factor in attempting to evaluate significance, particularly with respect to HLA class I antigens because of the large number of phenotypes. Preliminary follow-up studies (Connor *et al.* 1993) have shown that patients with early cervical cancers which have down-regulated HLA class I have a poorer clinical outcome. If this is the result of immunoselection then an association with particular HLA polymorphisms should be apparent. However the serological definition of HLA antigens does not discriminate among alleles with the same specificity as the T cell repertoire. As more HLA alleles are sequenced, more information on the rules for binding peptides will become apparent and any association with disease more explicable. It is possible that HLA-B locus products (polymorphisms) may be more relevant for presentation of target peptides than HLA-A locus products. This might explain the high frequency of HLA-B locus down-regulation seen in both premalignant and malignant lesions of the cervix in the study of Cromme *et al.* (1993a). One interesting possibility is that such locus specific HLA class I loss may be the result of the differential requirement for a functional peptide transporter system for surface expression of HLA-B compared to HLA-A allelic products. The expression of the TAP gene products and related systems should be a focus for future studies.

The role of HLA in susceptibility to HPV-related cancer is strongly supported by the observation that regression and progression of cottontail rabbit PV-associated papillomas in rabbits are linked respectively to the MHC-DR and -DQ genotype of the animals (Han *et al.* 1992). Such an association occurring in cervical HPV 16 infection could explain why some HPVI and CIN lesions persist or progress whilst others regress. However, it is possible that cervical disease association with HLA may reflect polymorphism of non-class I or II genes within the MHC, for example the TAP genes (Kelly *et al.* 1992). In rats, polymorphism at the TAP loci influences the spectrum of peptides presented by class I (Powis *et al.* 1992). However, it should be remembered that in humans, the extent of TAP polymorphism is much more limited, and there is no evidence to date that human TAP polymorphism regulates peptide presentation.

9.6   Implications for immunological intervention

It remains a possibility that certain HLA antigens may influence the development of squamous cell carcinoma of the cervix. Many immune responses are controlled by the genes of the MHC and loss of HLA class I expression has been demonstrated in a significant proportion of SCC while the majority, in contrast to normal cervical squamous epithelium, express HLA class II antigens. There are clearly several MHC factors contributing to the overall immune response to these tumours and to the viral agents that have been implicated in their etiology.

It is likely that the class I down-regulated phenotype is heterogeneous in origin and we cannot yet exclude that in some cases this is a consequence of HPV gene expression. The absence of HLA class I expression from whatever means would be expected to interfere directly with T cell recognition of target antigens. Thus any therapeutic immunization versus

HPV oncogene products may not be effective in targeting cytotoxic T cells to the cervical tumour cells. The possibility that the observed class I changes are late events reflecting the immunoselection of subpopulations of cells with immunological advantage cannot be ruled out. In considering treatment of premalignant disease by immunization versus HPV, the lack of class I changes seen in premalignant lesions must be confirmed in larger numbers of lesions that have or would be likely to progress to invasive cancer. Likewise it is necessary to consider the possible negative influences of the up-regulated HLA class II expression in CIN and SCC including induction of anergy in HPV specific T cells. In principle, prophylactic vaccination to HPV is feasible but demands much work to determine which HPV types, target antigens, and immunization routes would be likely to be effective. The relevance of specific requirements of eliciting mucosal immunity must be carefully considered. Whether HPV is found in a latent state like EBV might profoundly influence the adoption of such a strategy. Finally who is going to pay to immunize whom in which populations?

Acknowlegement

The authors are supported by the Cancer Research Campaign.

References

Bal, V., McIndoe, A., Denton, G., Hudson, D., Lombardi, G., and Lamb, J. (1990). Antigen presentation by keratinocytes induces tolerance in human T cells. *European Journal of Immunology*, 20, 1893–7.

Bartholomew, J., Tinsley, J., and Stern, P. L. (1994). *MHC expression in HPV-associated cervical cancer*. Cambridge University Press, in press.

Bjorkman, P. J., Saper, M. A., Samraoui, W. S., Bennett, J. L., Strominger, J. L., and Wiley, D. C. (1987). The foreign antigen binding site and T cell recognition regions of class I histocompatibility antigens. *Nature*, 329, 506–12.

Burke, F., Naylor, M. S., Davies, B., and Balkwill, F. (1993). The cytokine wall chart. *Immunology Today*, 14, 165–70.

Connor, M. E. and Stern, P. L. (1990). Loss of MHC class I expression in cervical carcinomas. *International Journal of Cancer*, 46, 1029–34.

Connor, M. E., Davidson, S. E., Stern, P. L., Arrand, J. R., and West, C. M. L. (1993). Evaluation of multiple biological parameters in cervical carcinoma: high macrophage infiltration in HPV-associated tumours. *International Journal of Gynecological Cancer*, 32, 103–9.

Couturier, J., Sastre-Garau, X., Schneider-Manoury, S., Labib, A., and Orth, G. (1991). Integration of papillomavirus DNA near myc genes in genital carcinomas and its consequences for proto-oncogene expression. *Journal of Virology*, 65, 4534–8.

Cox, J. H., Bennick, J. R., and Yewden, J. W. (1991). Retention of adenovirus E19 glycoprotein in the endoplasmic reticulum is essential to its ability to block antigen presentation. *Journal of Experimental Medicine*, **174**, 1629–37.

Cromme, F. V., Meijer, C. J. L. M., Snijders, P. J. F., Uyterlinde, A., Kenemans, P., Helmerhorst, T. *et al.* (1993a). Analysis of MHC class I and II expression in relation to presence of HPV genotypes in premalignant and malignant cervical lesions. *British Journal of Cancer*, **67**, 1372–80.

Cromme, F. V., Snidjers, P. J. F., van den Brule, A. J. C., Kenemans, P., Meijer, C. J. L. M., and Walboomers, J. M. M. (1993b). MHC class I expression in HPV 16 positive cervical carcinomas is post-transcriptionally controlled and independent from c-myc overexpression. *Oncogene*, in press.

Cromme, F. V., Airey, J., Heemels, M-T., Ploegh, H. L., Keating, P. J., Stern, P. L., Meijer, C. J. L. M. and Walboomers, J. M. M. (1994). Loss of transporter protein encoded by the TAP-1 gene, is highly correlated with loss of HLA expression in cervical carcinomas. *Journal of Experimental Medicine*, **179**, 335–40.

De Val, M., Hengel, H., Hacker, H., Hartlaub, U., Ruppert, T., Lucin, P. *et al.* (1992) Cytomegalovirus prevents antigen presentation by blocking the transport of peptide-loaded MHC class I molecules into the medial-Golgi compartment. *Journal of Experimental Medicine*, **176**, 729–38.

Drezen, J. M., Babinet, C., and Morello, D. (1993). Transcriptional control of MHC class I and beta-2 microglobulin genes *in vivo*. *Journal of Immunology*, **150**, 2805–13.

Garrido, F., and Ruiz-Cabello, F. (1991). MHC expression on human tumours —its relevance for local tumour growth and metastases. *Seminars in Cancer Biology*, **2**, 3–10.

Garrido, F., Cabrera, T., Concha, A., Glew, S. S., Ruiz-Cabello, F., and Stern, P. L. (1993). Natural history of HLA expression during tumour development. *Immunology Today*, **14**, 491–9.

Glew, S. S., Duggan-Keen, M., Cabrera, T., and Stern, P. L. (1992a). HLA class II antigen expression in human papillomavirus-associated cervical cancer. *Cancer Research*, **52**, 4009–16.

Glew, S. S., Stern, P. L., Davidson, J. A., and Dyer, P. A. (1992b). HLA antigens and cervical carcinoma. *Nature*, **356**, 22.

Glew, S. S., Connor, M. E., Snijders, P. J. F., Stanbridge, C. M., Buckley, C. H., Walboomers, J. M. M. *et al.* (1993a). HLA expression in preinvasive cervical neoplasia in relationship to human papillomavirus infection. *European Journal of Cancer*, **29A**, 1963–70.

Glew, S. S., Duggan-Keen, M., Ghosh, A. K., Ivinson, A., Sinnott, P., Davidson, J. *et al.* (1993b). Lack of association of HLA polymorphisms with HPV-related cervical cancer. *Human Immunology*, **37**, 157–64.

Han, R., Breitburd, F., Marche, P. N., and Orth, G. (1992). Linkage of regression and malignant conversions of rabbit papillomas to MHC class II genes. *Nature*, **356**, 66–8.

Harding, F. A., McArthur, J. G., Gross, J. A., Raulet, D. H., and Allison, J. P. (1992). CD28-mediated signalling co-stimulates murine T cells and prevents induction of anergy in T-cell clones. *Nature*, **356**, 607–9.

Helland, A., Borresen, A. L., Kaern, J., Ronningen, K. S., and Thorsby, E. (1992). HLA antigens and cervical carcinoma. *Nature*, **356**, 23.

Hughes, R. G., Norval, M., and Howie, S. M. (1988). Expression of major histocompatibility antigens by Langerhans cells in cervical intra-epithelial neoplasia. *Journal of Clinical Pathology*, **41**, 253–9.

Kelly, A., Powis, S. H., Kerr, L. A., Mockridge, I., Elliott, T., Bastin, J. *et al.* (1992). Assembly and function of the two ABC transporter proteins encoded in the human major histocompatibility complex. *Nature*, **355**, 641–4.

McIndoe, W. A., MacLean, M. R., and Jones, R. W. (1984). The invasive potential of carcinoma-in-situ of the cervix. *Obstetrics Gynecology*, **64**, 451–8.

Monaco, J. J. (1992). A molecular model of MHC class I-restricted antigen processing. *Immunology Today*, **13**, 173–8.

Neefjes, J. J. and Ploegh, H. L. (1988). Allele and locus-specific differences in cell surface expression and the association of HLA class I heavy chain with beta2-microglobulin: differential effects of inhibition of glycosylation on class I subunit association. *European Journal of Immunology*, **18**, 801–10.

Neefjes, J. J. and Pleogh, H. (1992). Intracellular transport of MHC class II molecules. *Immunology Today*, **13**, 179–83.

Nickoloff, B. J., Mitra, R. S., Green, J., Zheng, X-G, Shimizu, Y., Thompson, C. *et al.* (1993). Accessory cell function of keratinocytes for superantigens. *Journal of Immunology*, **150**, 2148–59.

Powis, S. J., Deverson, E. V., Coadwell, W. J., Ciruela, A., Huskisson, N. S., Smith, H. *et al.* (1992). Effect of polymorphism of an MHC-linked transporter on the peptides assembled in a class I molecule. *Nature*, **357**, 211–15.

Restifo, N. P., Esquivel, F., Kawakami, Y., Yewdell, J. W., Mule, J. J., Rosenberg, S. A. *et al.* (1993). Identification of human cancers deficient in antigen processing. *Journal of Experimental Medicine*, **177**, 265–72.

Rudensky, A. Y., Preston-Hurlburt, P., Hong, S. C., Barlow, A., and Janeway, C. A. (1991). Sequence analysis of peptides bound to MHC class II molecules. *Nature*, **353**, 622–7.

Schmidt, H., Gekeler, V., Haas, H. Engler-Blum, G., Steiert, I., Probst, H. *et al.* (1990). Differential regulation of HLA class I genes by interferon. *Immunogenetics*, **31**, 245–52.

Schneider, A., and Koutsky, L. (1992). Natural history and epidemiological features of genital HPV infection. In *The epidemiology of human papillomavirus and cervical cancer* (eds. N. Munoz, F. X. Bosch, K. V. Shah, and A. Meheus), Vol. 119, pp.23–52. International Agency for Research on Cancer, Lyon, France.

Schrier, P. I., Bernards, R., Vaessen, R. T. M. J., Houweling, A, and van der Erb, A. J. (1983). Expression of class I major histocompatibility complex antigens switched off by highly oncogenic adenovirus 12 in transformed rat cells. *Nature*, **311**, 750.

Springer, T. A. (1990). Adhesion receptors of the immune system. *Nature*, **346**, 425–34.

Townsend, A., Elliott, T., Cerundolo, V., Foster, L., Barber, B., and Tse, A. (1990). Assembly of MHC class I molecules analyzed *in vitro*. *Cell*, **62**, 285–95.

Versteeg, R., Kruse-Wolters, M., Plomp, A. C., van Leeuwen, A. A. D., Stam, N. J., Ploegh, H. L. *et al.* (1989). Suppression of class I human histocompatibility leukocyte antigen by c-myc is locus-specific. *Journal of Experimental Medicine*, **170**, 621–35.

Wank, R., and Thomssen, C. (1991). High risk of squamous cell carcinoma of the cervix for women with HLA-DQw3. *Nature*, **352**, 723–5.

Wank, R., Schendel, D. J., and Thomssen, C. (1992). HLA antigens and cervical carcinoma. *Nature*, **356**, 22–23.

10 Towards vaccines against papillomavirus

M. SAVERIA CAMPO

10.1 Papillomavirus is oncogenic

As already described elsewhere (Chapter 2), papillomaviruses induce a variety of lesions both in humans and in animals. Some papillomas, albeit benign, are themselves a clinical problem, such as laryngeal papillomas of children (Steinberg 1987) or penile papillomas of bulls (Jarrett 1985), and others are known to be a risk factor in the pathogenesis of cancer. In humans, papillomavirus infection of the genital tract can lead to squamous cell carcinoma particularly in the uterine cervix (zur Hausen 1991), and infection of the skin by certain virus types can develop into squamous cancer in immunosuppressed individuals (Orth 1987). In animals, the link between papillomavirus and cancer of the skin in rabbits, and of the urinary bladder and the upper alimentary canal in cattle, is well documented (Kreider 1980; Campo and Jarrett 1986; Campo *et al.* 1992).

10.2 Co-operation between virus and co-factors

Despite its undisputed involvement in malignancies, the virus is a necessary but not sufficient agent for the full development of cancer, and it is accepted that other factors, both extrinsic and intrinsic, play a pivotal role in the malignant progression of precancerous lesions. Indeed, involvement of cofactors is a characteristic of papillomavirus-linked cancers, but, while our understanding of the viral contribution to carcinogenesis has been significantly advanced in recent years with the identification of several papillomavirus transforming genes and some of their cellular targets (see Chapter 5), we still know relatively little concerning the interplay of chemical carcinogens with virus in tumour progression, particularly in humans. In cottontail rabbits, the cottontail rabbit papillomavirus (CRPV) induces papillomas, 25 per cent of which can progress to cancer. In domestic rabbits, however, up to 75 per cent of the lesions can progress to cancer in a shorter time, pointing to the genetic constitution of the host as one of the factors in malignant progression (Kreider 1980). In addition, application of tar and/or methylcholantrene to papillomas greatly accelerates their conversion to cancer (Rous and Friedewald 1944), as shown in one of the earliest demonstrations of synergism between virus and chemicals.

In cattle, carcinogenesis of the alimentary canal and of the urinary bladder is linked to infection by bovine papillomavirus (BPV) type 4 and type 2 respectively, and to the presence of bracken fern in the diet (Campo and Jarrett 1986; Campo *et al.* 1992). Bracken fern contains immuno-suppressants and mutagens (reviewed by Jackson *et al.* 1993) and both classes of compounds are needed for malignant progression of the neo-plastic lesions (Campo and Jarrett 1986). Immunosuppression allows the spread and the life-long persistence of the infection and the mutagens induce additional genetic damages to the infected cell. The flavonoid quercetin, one of the most potent mutagens in bracken, synergizes with BPV-4 in inducing malignant cell transformation *in vitro* (Pennie and Campo 1992).

In humans, the co-factors are less well identified. Inherited immuno-deficiency is a predisposing factor in the conversion of skin warts to squamous cell cancer in patients with *Epidermodysplasia verruciformis* (*EV*), and malignant progression is observed more frequently in areas exposed to sunlight, implicating UV radiation as an additional factor (Orth 1987). In the case of cervical cancer, the identity of co-factors is rather nebulous: number of sexual partners, age at first intercourse, infection with herpes simplex type 2 (HSV-2), and/or other sexually transmitted pathogens, smok-ing, local and/or systemic immunodeficiency, all seem to play a role, alongside certain human papillomavirus (HPV) types, primarily HPV-16, in the pathogenesis of the disease (reviewed by Brinton 1992). The possible involvement of HSV-2 has not been excluded (DiPaolo, *et al.* 1990). Smoking provides a source of carcinogens and it has been shown that the cervical mucous of smokers is mutagenic (Holly *et al.* 1986) and this cor-relates with a higher level of DNA adducts in cervical biopsies (Phillips and Ni She 1993). In addition smoking elicits marked alteration in the immune system, including reduction of IgA, IgG, and IgM concentrations and suppression of T cell function (Holt 1987).

10.3   The role of the immune system in the control of papillomavirus infection

One constant in the diseases described above is an impairment of immune functions, providing evidence that the host's immune system plays a major role in controlling the course of papillomavirus infection. Immuno-deficiency or immunosuppression, whether hereditary, iatrogenic, or ac-quired, permits both virus and infected cells to evade immunosurveillance, with the consequent development and persistence of the premalignant lesions and the development of cancer. In immunocompetent hosts papillomavirus infection is self-limiting in the great majority of cases and the lesions regress spontaneously.

Wart regression is systemic; when several warts are present, the regression of one wart is accompanied by regression of the others. However, regression is also wart-type specific; for instance, common warts do not regress in patients with regressing flat warts. As different types of warts are caused by different HPV types (De Villiers 1989), the specificity of regression suggests that the rejection mechanism operates against type-specific viral antigens.

Several lines of circumstantial evidence indicate that regression of papillomavirus-induced lesions is due to cell-mediated immunity (CMI) and not to a humoral antibody response. The presence of circulating anti-papillomavirus antibodies, including neutralizing ones, does not induce tumour regression, and disorders of humoral immunity do not result in increased susceptibility to papillomavirus infection (Lutzner 1985). In contrast, infiltrates of mononuclear cells, B- and T-lymphocytes, occur in spontaneously regressing skin warts and genital condylomas in humans and in cattle. Immunocompetent cells are present also in cervical lesions of HPV origin and in oral lesions with a possible HPV etiology (for references relevant to immune cell infiltrates, see Campo 1991).

Further support to the involvement of CMI in the regression of papillomavirus lesions is provided by the increased susceptibility to papillomavirus infection of individuals with either genetic or acquired cell-mediated immunodeficiencies, and by the increased persistance and incidence of neoplastic progression of warts in these subjects (reviewed by Benton *et al.* 1992). A well-known example of malignant conversion of papillomavirus-induced lesions in individuals with genetic cell-mediated immunodeficiency is provided by EV patients who suffer disseminated long-lasting warty lesions which frequently progress to cancer, especially in sun-exposed skin (Orth 1987). Similar phenomena are observed in renal transplant patients immunosuppressed as a result of therapy, who present an increased incidence of both skin warts and cervical intra-epithelial neoplasia (CIN), accompanied by a reduction in intra-epithelial T-cells in CIN lesions (reviewed by Benton *et al.* 1992). Significantly increased evidence of cervical and anorectal HPV infection has been documented in individuals with symptomatic human immunodeficiency virus (HIV) infection (reviewed by Judson 1992), pointing again to the role of the immune system in controlling papillomavirus infection.

This situation is reminiscent of the etiology of alimentary canal cancer in cattle. Papillomas of the upper alimentary canal spread, persist, and progress with high frequency to squamous cell carcinomas in animals immunosuppressed either naturally or experimentally (Campo and Jarrett 1986).

10.4   Vaccination against papillomavirus

In principle, reduction of the incidence of papillomavirus-linked cancers could be achieved by either intervening against the co-factors or against the virus. Elimination of co-factors is problematic. They are still ill-defined in the case of cervical cancer, and even when they have been identified, as is the case for smoking, it is not easy to induce behavioural changes in a population at risk. Therefore, it is conceptually easier, at least for this writer, to envisage strategies directed against the virus itself or against the premalignant lesions it induces. Discussion on antiviral drugs is beyond the scope of this chapter and thus only the prospects for vaccination will be considered.

Both in human and in veterinary medicine there is a need for anti-papillomavirus vaccines in the treatment of recalcitrant warts and in prevention of malignant progression. The vaccines could be either conventionally prophylactic, designed to prevent infection, or therapeutic, if capable of inducing tumour rejection.

Knowledge of the host humoral and cell-mediated immune response against the infectious agents helps the design of more effective vaccines. Unfortunately, in the case of papillomaviruses, this knowledge is still fragmentary, despite rapid progress being made. Many aspects of papillomavirus research, and primarily the immunological ones, have been delayed by the limited amount of virus recoverable from some lesions, in particular from those of the cervix, and by the impossibility of growing *in vitro* the necessary quantities of virus, with resultant lack of reagents. The production of viral proteins both in bacteria and in eukaryotic cells and the use of synthetic peptides have circumvented this last problem and have allowed the ongoing analysis of the humoral and cellular immune response to papillomavirus infection (see Campo 1991 for relevant references). However, to complicate matters even further, papillomaviruses appear to elicit little if any immune response. This may relate to the fact that the virus infects keratinocytes and does not kill the infected cell. Infection may influence MHC class I or class II antigen expression which in turn may affect the recruitment of T-cells (see Chapters 8 and 9).

While investigations into human papillomavirus vaccines are at their beginning, vaccines against the animal papillomaviruses BPV and CRPV were already in use several decades ago (Campo 1991).

10.5   Animal papillomavirus vaccines

Animal models present many advantages over human ones. The most important and most obvious is the possibility of direct experimentation, which is, of course, unethical in human subjects. Contrary to the human case, the natural history of papillomavirus infection in animals is reasonably well known (Kreider 1980; Jarrett 1985); animals can be infected in controlled conditions and longitudinal studies can be pursued, both in the field of immunology (Jarrett *et al.* 1991; Okabayashi *et al.* 1991; Han *et al.* 1992) and in that of carcinogenesis (Campo and Jarrett 1986; Campo *et al.* 1992). Another advantage is given by the choice of studying either outbred individuals, such as rabbits and cattle, or inbred ones, such as mice, thus providing the opportunity of investigating the role of MHC in the immune response. Rabbits are small, easily manageable and relatively short-lived; experiments in rabbits tend to last from a few months to two years. Cattle, like humans, are big, long-lived and outbred; experiments in calves tend to last approximately from one to fifteen years. Mice do not need much description as experimental animals. They have proved invaluable in showing that the immune response to particular epitopes of HPV-16 is MHC restricted (see Chapters 8 and 9); on the other hand, the results obtained with mice have to be carefully evaluated in the light of the demonstration that the so-called 'public epitope' of HPV-16 E7, first identified in mice (Tindle *et al.* 1991), is not recognized by infected human subjects (Frazer and Tindle 1992), and may be specific to mice only. Mice are not naturally infected with HPV; indeed no papillomavirus has yet been isolated from mice in the wild, and the immune system of laboratory mice has no knowledge of HPV until experimental infection. On the contrary, in both cattle and rabbits, experiments are conducted with the host species natural pathogen: the host and the virus have co-evolved and adapted to each other and therefore the immunological response observed in experimental situations is likely to be meaningful and to reflect biological processes that occur naturally.

10.6 'Natural' vaccines

Early vaccines against BPV and CRPV were based on crude wart extracts. The BPV vaccines were only partially successful in preventing spread of papillomatosis through cattle herds, and the reasons responsible for their success or failure were not understood. We now know that at least six different papillomavirus types affect cattle, which are immunological distinct entities displaying little or no antigenic cross-reactivity. Thus, one possible reason for the failure of past experiments was that the vaccines were probably derived from tumours induced by a virus type different from the actual type causing the infection. This hypothesis has been confirmed by experimentation in cattle. Vaccination with purified BPV-2 or extracts from BPV-2-induced papillomas protected animals from infection with the same virus, but not from infection with other BPVs. Vaccinated animals had high titres of serum neutralizing antibodies, widely believed to be responsible for eliciting immunity. Vaccines based on BPV-2-transformed cells, in which only the early (non-structural) but not the late (structural) viral proteins are synthesized were not successful, supporting the notion that neutralizing antibodies are directed at superficial epitopes on strucural proteins. Primary references on natural vaccines against animal papillomaviruses can be found in Campo (1991).

10.7 'Recombinant' vaccines: Late proteins

The virion of papillomavirus is made up of two proteins; L1, the major capsid protein which constitutes approximately 75 per cent of the virion, and L2, the minor one which makes up the remaining 25 per cent. The presence of neutralizing epitopes on the structural proteins has been confirmed by vaccination experiments which use individual viral proteins, usually in the form of a fusion with a bacterial protein. This is achieved by molecularly cloning the L1 or L2 gene in a prokaryotic plasmid, usually 3′ to a bacterial gene so that the viral component is transcribed and translated as a read-through product. The L1 gene of BPV-1 and the L1 and L2 genes of BPV-2 have been cloned and expressed in bacteria as β-galactosidase fusion proteins (Pilacinski *et al.* 1986; Jarrett *et al.* 1991); the L1 and L2 genes of CRPV have been cloned and expressed as λ-cII or trpE fusion products (Christensen *et al.* 1991; Lin *et al.* 1992), and the L2 gene of BPV-4 has been cloned and expressed as glutathione-S-transferase (GST) fusions (Campo *et al.* 1993). The structural genes of CRPV have also been molecularly cloned in vaccinia vectors, and the resulting recombinant vaccina viruses have been used as live vaccines (Lin *et al.* 1992). Whether the vaccine was based on recombinant protein or recombinant vaccinia virus, L1 was found in all cases to protect vaccinated animals from infection (Table 10.1; Pilacinski *et al.* 1986; Jarrett *et al.* 1991; Lin *et al.* 1992) and the L1-vaccinated animals had high titres of serum neutralizing antibodies (Jarrett *et al.* 1991; Lin *et al.* 1992). Thus, L1 encodes neutralizing epitopes and at least some of the epitopes are not conformational.

Vaccination with L2 seems to achieve different effects with different viruses. Vaccination of rabbits with the L2 protein of CRPV protected the animals from further challenge. The protected animals had low titres of serum neutralizing antibodies (Table 10.1; Christensen *et al.* 1991; Lin *et al.* 1992). Vaccination of cattle with the L2 protein of BPV-2 did not prevent infection but induced early regression of established warts (Fig. 10.1). Although the vaccinated animals had high titre antibodies against L2, these were not neutralizing (Table 10.1; Jarrett *et al.* 1991). Heavy infiltrates of immune cells were present in the regressing warts, and, although the nature of the cellular immune response was not further defined,

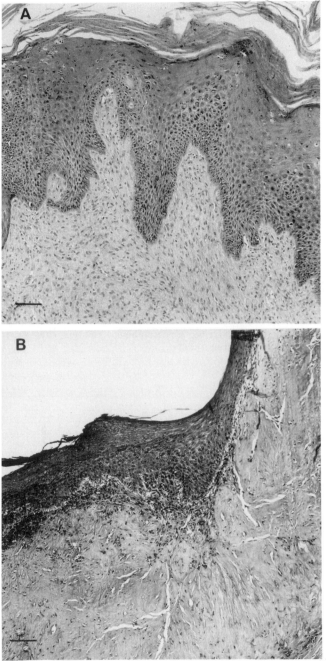

Fig. 10.1 Regression of skin papillomas in cattle vaccinated with BPV-2 L2. A: H & E stained histological section of a skin papilloma. B: regressing skin papilloma; note the infiltrate of immune cells in the subepithelial dermis. Bar represents 10 μM.

Table 10.1 Recombinant papillomavirus vaccines

Vaccine	Protection
Structural proteins	
BPV-1 L1[a]	Protection
BPV-2 L1[a]	Protection—neutralizing Abs
BPV-2 L2[a]	Rejection—no neutralizing Abs—CMI
BPV-4 L2[a]	Protection
CRPV L1[a,b]	Protection—high titre neutralizing Abs
CRPV L2[a]	Protection—low titre neutralizing Abs
Early proteins	
BPV-4 E7[a]	Growth retardation and tumour rejection
BPV-1 E5[b,c]	
BPV-1 E6[b,c]	Growth retardation and tumour rejection
BPV-1 E7[b,c]	
HPV-16 E6[b,c]	Growth retardation, tumour rejection,
HPV-16 E7[b,c]	graft rejection

a recombinant protein vaccine; b recombinant vaccinia virus vaccine;
c experiments performed in rodents

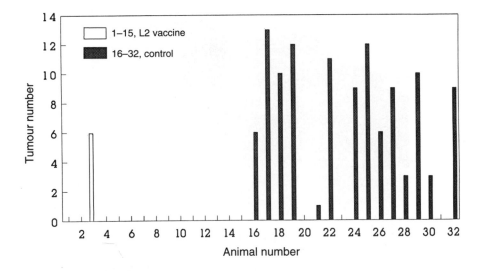

Fig. 10.2 Protection from infection in cattle vaccinated with BPV-4 L2. Only one animal in the vaccinated group developed alimentary canal papillomas, compared with fourteen out of seventeen animals in the control group.

it appeared that L2 could elicit the activation of the cellular effector arm of the immune system. Vaccination of cattle with the L2 protein of BPV-4 afforded virtually complete protection from further virus challenge (Fig. 10.2; Table 10.1; Campo *et al.* 1993). It is not yet known whether protection is due to a virus neutralization event, as is the case for CRPV L2, or to a very early cell-mediated immune response directed against the infected cell; in this case BPV-4 L2 would operate through the same immunological mechanisms of BPV-2 L2 but on a different timescale.

10.8 'Recombinant' vaccines: Early proteins

E6 and E7 are the major oncoproteins of HPV-16 (see Chapter 5). BPV-4 is unusual in its lack of an E6 gene; E7 is its major transforming protein *in vitro* (Jackson and Campo 1992), and is expressed throughout the different developmental stages of alimentary canal papillomas (R. Anderson and M.S. Campo, unpublished observations), pointing to its importance for the maintenance of the proliferative state also *in vivo*. The functions of the papillomavirus oncoproteins have been described in detail in Chapters 2 and 5. The pivotal role of E6 and E7 in cell transformation has lead to speculation that these proteins may behave immunologically

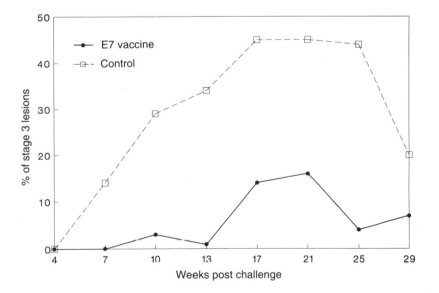

Fig. 10.3 Growth retardation and regression of alimentary canal papillomas in cattle vaccinated with BPV-4 E7. In the vaccinated group, less than 20 per cent of the papillomas developed to stage 3, compared with approximately 50 per cent in the control group.

like SV40 T antigen (Anderson *et al.* 1988) or adenovirus E1A (Kast *et al.* 1989) and be targets for a cellular immune response which would result in tumour regression. This hypothesis has been proved true in cattle. In cattle vaccinated with BPV-4 E7 as a β-gal fusion protein, the growth of papillomas is retarded and the tumours are rejected earlier than in control animals (Fig. 10.3; Table 10.1; Campo *et al.* 1993). In contrast, vaccination with E2, another early protein, is ineffective. Vaccination with E7 therefore provides successful therapy for papillomas in a natural animal model.

In a rat system also the early proteins of BPV-1 were found to be partially effective. In this case the early ORFs of BPV-1 were cloned in vaccinia viruses, and the live recombinant vaccinia viruses were assessed for their ability to elicit anti-tumour immunity in rats seeded with BPV-1 transformed oncogenic syngeneic cells. Increased latency periods of tumour development were observed in some of the rats vaccinated with recombinants expressing E5, E6, or E7 (Table 10.1; Meneguzzi *et al.* 1990). E2 was found to be ineffective, as in cattle.

10.9   Immune response to vaccine E7

Vaccination of cattle with E7 is accompanied by both a humoral and a cellular immune response to the vaccine. Both responses appear much earlier and have a greater amplitude in the vaccinated animals than in the control calves. Indeed, some of the control animals never developed detectable antibodies to E7 throughout the course of the experiment (Chandrechud *et al.* 1994). Vaccine E7 is therefore successfully presented to both effector arms of the immune system, while viral E7 is poorly presented. This may explain the efficacy of the vaccine. The immunodominant B- and T-cell epitopes encoded by E7 have been mapped to the termini of the protein. B1 and T1 map to the amino terminus and B2 and T2 to the carboxyl terminus (Chandrechud *et al.* 1994; G. McGarvie, unpublished observations). Two interesting observations derive from these results. First, B- and T-cell epitopes map in the same regions of E7; second, both these regions of BPV-4 E7 have amino acid and functional homology to HPV-16 E7 (Jackson and Campo 1992) and the same areas in HPV-16 E7 have been shown to contain B- and T-cell epitopes (see Chapters 7 and 8). The immunological homology between conserved areas of BPV-4 and HPV-16 E7 proteins leads to the prediction that the latter will be effective in promoting tumour regression in humans.

10.10   'HPV-16 vaccines'

Clearly, the structural proteins L1 and L2 and the transforming proteins E6 and E7 of different animal papillomaviruses elicit the appropriate immune response to induce immunity from infection and retardation of tumour growth and tumour rejection respectively, thus strongly encouraging the view that vaccination is also possible in human subjects. The success obtained against the mucosal virus BPV-4 is particularly remarkable and of special relevance to the possible use of vaccines against genital HPVs. Vaccination against papillomavirus and papillomavirus-induced tumours in human patients is not a novel idea. Almost fifty years ago, vaccination for warts and condylomas was performed using both autologous and heterologous phenolic extracts of warts and condylomas; approximately 80 per cent of the patients were reported as either completely or partially cured. More recently, autogenous vaccines made from extracts of laryngeal papillomas or genital condylomas were shown to be effective in approximately 50 per cent and 80 per cent of the cases respectively (reviewed by Campo 1991). The nature of the target antigen was not known, but there is recent circumstantial evidence that it may have been the E7 oncoprotein. In experimental systems HPV-16 E7 behaves immunologically like E7 of BPV-4 and BPV-1, and may thus provide the means to an effective therapeutic vaccine. Vaccination of rats or mice with live recombinant vaccinia viruses containing the HPV-16 E7 gene caused growth retardation and partial regression of tumours induced by syngeneic oncogenic HPV-16 transformed cells (Table 10.1; Meneguzzi *et al.* 1991; Chen *et al.* 1991). In the mouse system, it has been shown that tumour regression is due to the activation of E7-specific CD8[+] cytotoxic T-lymphocytes (CTLs) (Chen *et al.* 1991). In this system therefore, E7 appears to act as a classical tumour rejection antigen. However, in a similar system which exploits the grafting of HPV-16 transformed but non-malignant mouse keratinocytes in syngeneic mice, early rejection of the graft is accompanied by measurable delayed type hypersensitivity (DTH) response against the E7 protein (McLean *et al.* 1993). The response is mediated by CD4[+] lymphocytes, with no involvement of CTLs. The experimental induction of a DTH response is of considerable importance, as such response is observed in the spontaneous regression of cutaneous and genital warts in man (Benton *et al.* 1992; M. Stanley, personal communication). In fact, the presence of E7-specific CTLs during tumour regression in a natural host is still an open question. No CTLs have yet been identified in regressor calves vaccinated with BPV-4 E7 or in HPV-16 infected human subjects, and CTLs involvement is not apparent in graft, as opposed to tumour, rejection in mice.

Whatever the detailed immunological mechanisms, on the basis of the success obtained in animal models, L1 and L2 appear to be the best candidates for prophylactic vaccination, and E7 for therapeutic vaccination also in humans. It is only a matter of time before these proteins, or their genes, enter clinical trials.

10.11   Considerations for future human papillomavirus vaccines

It has been noted that all the papillomavirus proteins used as vaccines in the cattle and rabbit systems have so far been fused with a bacterial protein. The immunological efficacy of viral proteins free of bacterial constituents has not yet been tested. The identity of the bacterial moiety does not seem to be crucial as β-gal, GST, trpE, or λ-cII fusions have all been used in different laboratories with excellent results. It is, however, possible that the bacterial portion of the vaccine acting as a hapten provides a strong stimulus for the immune system, without which the vaccine would be less effective. If this were the case, it would have profound implications for the development of human vaccines, as bacterial fusion proteins are not considered appropriate for human use. Viral protein vaccines, without a bacterial component, will soon be tried in the cattle system. Another question arising in the design of HPV protein vaccines concerns the source of the proteins. The viral proteins will have to be made in expression systems compatible with human usage. Bacterially expressed proteins, even if not in fusion form, are deemed unsuitable because of the possible presence of endotoxins in the preparation. On the other hand, yeast is already being used as a source of hepatitis B virus protein for vaccination purposes and therefore should be equally successful as a source of papillomavirus proteins.

The nature of the viral proteins is also a subject of concern. Anxiety is sometimes expressed about the safety of using the oncoprotein E7 as a vaccine. Although there is no documented reason for such a concern, it may be that a mutant E7, defective for cell transformation, will be more acceptable as a vaccine, provided it retains its immunological characteristics. In this context it is noteworthy that the immunodominant T-cell epitopes in BPV-4 and HPV 16 E7 map to the $p105^{Rb}$ binding domain and to the second cys-x-x-cys motif, both essential regions for the transforming functions of the protein. It remains to be seen if mutations of these or other domains can be found which abolish the oncogenic potential of the protein without destroying its T cell epitopes as well.

A more difficult question to answer concerns which sections of the population to target for vaccination. For full prophylaxis, once effective and safe HPV vaccines are developed, it may be desirable to vaccinate the whole population at a young age, as is the case, for example, for polio or measles vaccines. A programme of prophylactic vaccination, even if starting in the near future, would not affect those sectors of the population currently at risk. These could be targeted and administered either a prophylactic or a therapeutic vaccine.

Despite these uncertainties, the striking success of the recent vaccination trials in animals strongly support the optimistic prediction that in the relatively near future vaccines will be available against the most problematic or potentially dangerous forms of papillomatosis in humans.

10.12   Summary

As papillomavirus is one of the major causative factors of cervical cancer, vaccines that eliminated papillomavirus infection would result in the eventual decrease of the incidence of the disease. In principle two different types of vaccine can be envisaged: prophylactic vaccines, which would elicit virus neutralizing antibodies and would prevent infection, and therapeutic vaccines which would induce regression of established lesions before progression to malignancy takes place. The research on vaccines against human papillomavirus (HPV) is hampered by the difficulties encountered in growing the virus in tissue culture and by the unacceptable nature of experimentation in humans. However, effective prophylactic vaccines, both natural and genetically engineered, have been developed against bovine papillomaviruses (BPVs) and cottontail rabbit papillomavirus (CRPV). The success obtained with the animal models supports the optimistic prediction that in the relatively near future vaccines will be available against the most problematic or potentially dangerous forms of papillomatosis in humans.

Acknowledgements

Many thanks are due to my collaborators, past and present, who have contributed to the work presented here; to the colleagues who have given me access to their unpublished data; to Dr John Wyke for critical review of the manuscript. Apologies are due to all those authors whose primary work could not be cited because of space restriction. Some of the ideas expressed in this chapter have already appeared in Campo (1991). My work is financed by the Cancer Research Campaign and I am a CRC Fellow.

References

Anderson, R. W., Tevethia, M. J., Kalderon, D., Smith, A. E., and Tevethia, S. S. (1988). Fine mapping of two distinct antigenic sites on SV40 T antigen reactive with SV40-specific cytotoxic T-cell clones by using SV40 deletion mutants. *Journal of Virology*, **62**, 285–96.

Benton, C., Shahidullah, H., and Hunter, J. A. A. (1992). Human papillomavirus in the immunosuppressed. *Papillomavirus Report*, **3**, 23–6.

Brinton, L. A. (1992). Epidemiology of cervical cancer—overview. In *The epidemiology human papillomavirus and cervical cancer* (eds. N. Munoz, F. X.

Bosch, K. V. Shah, and A. Meheus), pp. 3–23. IARC Scientific Publications No. 119.

Campo, M. S. (1991). Vaccination against papillomavirus. *Cancer Cells*, 3, 421–6.

Campo, M. S. and Jarrett, W. F. H. (1986). Papillomavirus infection in cattle: Viral and chemical cofactors in naturally occurring and experimental induced tumours. *Ciba Foundation Symposium*, 120, 117–35.

Campo, M. S., Jarrett, W. F. H., Barron, R., O'Neil, B. W., and Smith, K. T. (1992). Association of bovine papillomavirus type 2 and bracken fern with bladder cancer in cattle. *Cancer Research*, 52, 1–7.

Campo, M. S., Grindlay, G. J., O'Neil, B. W., Chandrachud, L. M., McGarvie, G. M., and Jarrett, W. F. H. (1993). Prophylactic and therapeutic vaccination against a mucosal papillomavirus. *Journal of General Virology*, 74, 945–53.

Chandrechud, L. M. O'Neil, B. W. Jarrett, W. F. H., Grindlay, G. J., McGarvie, G. M., and Campo, M. S. (1994). Humoral immune response to the E7 protein of bovine papillomavirus type 4, and identification of B-cell epitopes *Virology*, 199 (in press).

Chen, L., Thomas, E. K., Hu, S-L., Hellstrom, I., and Hellstrom, K. E. (1991). Human papillomavirus type 16 nucleoprotein E7 is a tumour rejection antigen. *Proceedings of National Academy of Sciences (USA)*, 88, 110–14.

Christensen, N. D., Kreider, J. W., Kan, N. C., and DiAngelo, S. L. (1991). The open reading frame L2 of cottontail rabbit papillomavirus contains antibody-inducing neutralizing epitopes. *Virology*, 181, 572–579.

De Villiers, E-M. (1989). Heterogeneity of the human papillomavirus group. *Journal of Virology*, 63, 4898–903.

Di Paolo, J. A., Woodworth, C. D., Popescu, N. C. Koval, D. L., Lopez, J. V. and Doniges, J. (1990) HSV-2 induced tumorigenicity in HPV-16 immortalized human genital keratinocytes. *Virology*, 177, 777–9.

Frazer, I. H. and Tindle, R. W. (1992). Cell-mediated immunity to papillomaviruses. *Papillomavirus Report*, 3, 53–8.

Han, R., Breitburd, F., Marche, P. N., and Orth, G. (1992). Linkage of regression and malignant conversion of rabbit viral papillomas to MHC class II genes. *Nature*, 356, 66–8.

Holly, E. A., Petrakis, N. L., Friend, N. F., Sarles, D. L., Lee, R. E., and Flander, L. B. (1986). Mutagenic mucus in the cervix of smokers. *Journal of the National Cancer Institute*, 76, 983–6.

Holt, P. G. (1987). Immune and inflammatory function in cigarette smokers. *Thorax*, 42, 241–9.

Jackson, M. E. and Campo, M. S. (1992). Bovine papillomaviruses. *Papillomavirus Report*, 3, 91–4.

Jackson, M. E., Campo, M. S., and Gaukroger, J. M. (1993). Cooperation between papillomavirus and chemical cofactors in oncogenesis. *Critical Reviews in Oncogenesis*, 3, in press.

Jarrett, W. F. H. (1985). The natural history of bovine papillomavirus infection. *Advances in Viral Oncology*, 5, 83–102.

Jarrett, W. F. H., Smith, K. T., O'Neil, B. W., Gaukroger, J. M., Chandrachud, L. M., Grindlay, G. J. *et al.* (1991). Studies on vaccination against papillomaviruses: Prophylactic and therapeutic vaccination with recombinant structural proteins. *Virology*, 184, 33–42.

Judson, F. N. (1992). Interactions between human papillomavirus and human immunodeficiency virus. In *The epidemiology of human papillomavirus and cervical cancer* (eds. N. Munoz, F. X. Bosch, K. V. Shah and A. Meheus), pp. 199–207. IARC Scientific Publications No. 119.

Kreider, J. W. (1980). Neoplastic progression of the Shope rabbit papilloma. In *Viruses in naturally occurring cancers*, (eds. M. Essex, G. Todaro and H. zur Hausen), pp. 283–99. CSH Laboratory Press.

Kast, W. M., Offringa, R., Peters, P. J., Voordouw, A. C., Meloen, R. H., Van der Eb, A. J. *et al.* (1989). Eradication of adenovirus E1-induced tumours by E1A-specific cytotoxic T-lymphocytes. *Cell*, **59**, 603–14.

Lin, Y-L., Borenstein, L. A., Selvakumar, R., Ahmed, R., and Wettstein, F. O. (1992). Effective vaccination against papilloma development by immunization with L1 or L2 structural proteins of cottontail rabbit papillomavirus. *Virology*, **187**, 612–19.

Lutzner, M. A. (1985). Papillomavirus lesions in immunodepression and immuno-suppression. *Clinics in Dermatology*, **3**, 165–9.

McLean, C. S., Sterling, J. S., Mowat, J., Nash, A. A., and Stanley, M. A. (1993). Delayed type hypersensitivity response to the human papillomavirus type 16 protein in a mouse model. *Journal of General Virology*, **74**, 239–45.

Meneguzzi, G., Kieny, M. P., Lecocq, J-P., Chambin, P., Cuzin, F., and Lathe, R. (1990). Vaccinia recombinants expressing early bovine papillomavirus proteins: retardation of BPV-1 tumour development. *Vaccine*, **8**, 199–204.

Meneguzzi, G., Cerni, C., Kieny, M. P., and Lathe, R. (1991). Immunization against human papillomavirus type 16 tumour cells with recombinant vaccinia viruses expressing E6 and E7. *Virology*, **181**, 62–9.

Okabayashi, M., Angell, M. G., Christensen, N. D., and Kreider, J. W. (1991). Morphometric analysis and identification of infiltrating leukocytes in regressing and progressing Shope rabbit papillomas. *International Journal of Cancer*, **49**, 919–23.

Orth, G. (1987). Epidermodysplasia verruciformis. In *The papovaviridae*, (eds. N. P. Salzman and P. M. Howley), Vol. 2, pp. 199–243. Plenum Press.

Pennie, W. D. and Campo, M. S. (1992). Synergism between bovine papilloma-virus type 4 and the flavonoid quercetin in cell transformation *in vitro*. *Virology*, **190**, 861–5.

Phillips, D. H. and Ni She M. (1993). Smoking-related DNA adducts in human cervical biopsies. In *Postlabelling methods for the detection of DNA damage* (eds. D. H. Phillips, M. Castegnaro, and H. Bartsch), pp. 327–30. IARC Scientific Publications.

Pilachinski, W. P., Glassman, D.L, Glassman, K. F., Reed, D. E., Lum, M. A., Marshall, R. F. *et al.* (1986). Immunization against bovine papillomavirus infection. *Ciba Foundation Symposium*, **120**, 136–48.

Rous, P. and Fricdewald, W. F. (1944). The effect of chemical carcinogens on virus-induced rabbit papillomas. *Journal of Experimental Medicine*, **79**, 511–49.

Steinberg, B. M. (1987). Laryngeal papillomas. Clinical aspects and *in vitro* studies. In *The papovaviridae* (eds. N. P. Saltzman and P. M. Howley), Vol.2, pp. 265–92. Plenum Press.

Tindle, R. W., Fernando, G. J., Sterling, J. C., and Frazer, I. H. (1991). A "public" T-helper epitope of the E7 transforming protein of human papilloma-virus 16 provides cognate help for several E7 B-cell epitopes from cervical cancer-associated human papillomavirus genotypes. *Proceedings of the National Institute of Sciences (USA)*, **88**, 5887–91.

zur Hausen, H. (1991). Human papillomaviruses in the pathogenesis of anogenital cancer. *Virology*, **184**, 9–13.

11 Immunological aspects of cutaneous warts

HUW DAVIES

11.1 Introduction

Much effort is being devoted to understanding the immunobiology of human papillomaviruses. Owing to the overwhelming experimental and epidemiological evidence to implicate the 'high risk' HPV types (notably, HPV 16 and 18) in the development of cancer of the cervix, much of this research effort is focused on the high-risk group. The rationale is two-fold. Firstly, the identification of naturally occurring immune responses will have implications in the design of vaccination strategies. Thus, the kinds of responses and the target viral antigens associated with natural immunity may allow us to elicit particular kinds of responses known to have protective value. It must be pointed out, however, that in no case has a full understanding of naturally occurring protective responses to a particular pathogen been required to develop any of the successful human or animal vaccines that exist. A second, and a perhaps more important, rationale for understanding immunity comes from the imminent phase 1 trials of a variety of HPV 16 vaccines to be conducted in patients. It will be essential that the reagents, technologies, and expertise are in place to determine the nature and efficacy of the response elicited. In particular, it will be important to know whether such vaccines stimulate HPV-specific cell-mediated or humoral responses, whether such responses are systemic or site (particularly cervix) specific, and the longevity of the response.

In this discussion I will examine the unique opportunities the benign cutaneous and mucosal HPVs offer for immunological study. In short, benign warts are overt and spontaneously regress, and although difficult to treat, rarely life threatening. These features facilitate the identification of people likely to have mounted protective responses to HPVs, in addition to representing a suitable lesion for testing immunotherapies. In contrast, individuals who may be protected from high-risk HPV infection are more difficult to find. Such lesions often go unnoticed, requiring colposcopy to visualize, thereby making prior histories and incidences of spontaneous regression almost impossible to establish. Moreover, the urgency to treat high-risk lesions by surgery will complicate therapeutic trials. The opportunities offered by the study of benign warts may also help resolve an apparent paradox concerning immunity to high-risk HPV.

11.2   The paradox

Without doubt, understanding immunity to high-risk genital HPVs has presented us with problems. These have been due largely to the necessity to develop valid synthetic antigens. Recent advances in the production of HPV in organotypic culture *in vitro* (Meyers *et al.* 1992) could revolutionize the approaches taken to elicit and detect immune responses to HPV in the near future. At the time of writing, however, the full potential of infectious virus is yet to be realized, and synthetic antigens remain the most convenient reagents for immunological study. These are now being designed with ever-increasing levels of sophistication and ingenuity. In particular, synthetic HPV particles, which self-assemble from recombinant capsid proteins (Zhou *et al.* 1992, 1993; Kirnbauer *et al.* 1992; Hagensee *et al.* 1993; Rose *et al.* 1993), will allow us to re-evaluate the mass of serological data collected hitherto using non-native capsid antigens. In parallel, recombinant proteins and synthetic peptides are proving useful for the stimulation of T cells and the mapping of epitopes recognized. However, synthetic reagents are not without their problems.

To date, studies in humans have been concerned with detecting naturally occurring responses to HPV. In other diseases, the mediators of specific immunity (antibodies, and proliferative or cytotoxic T cells) are widely used as indicators of past exposure to the aetiological agent, and synthetic re-agents have not hindered correlating responses with disease status. In contrast, most studies have shown that immune responses to high-risk HPV types can be detected in both symptomatic 'patients' and asymptomatic 'controls'. Equally puzzling is that some individuals from both groups also seem devoid of responses. Distinguishing an artifact associated with a synthetic reagent or with the assay conditions from a genuine presence (or absence) of a response to the virus is a major issue concerning HPV immunology. These observations have led to the suspicion that subclinical HPV infections are widespread within the population, that high-risk HPVs are not particularly immunogenic, or that high-risk HPVs may be trans-mitted by means other than sexual contact. As a consequence, the relative importance of cellular responses (cytotoxicity and inflammation) versus humoral responses (antibodies) in protection has not been defined. Pre-dictions can be made on the basis of what has been learned from other model viral systems. We might predict therefore that a secretory IgA response may act prophylactically to block infection of the cervical mucosa, whereas inflammatory or cytotoxic responses in the cervical epithelium would eliminate infected cells. These predictions form the framework for immunological investigations, but we must be aware of 'unfashionable' responses to HPV that may go unnoticed.

The major aims of immunological study therefore are to determine the immunogenicity of high-risk HPV (i.e., the ability to be recognized and to elicit a response from the immune system, whether naturally or by vaccination), to correlate responses with disease regression or progression, and to identify protective responses. Two criteria must be satisfied: (1) that the assay and the response thus measured is HPV specific, and (2) the status of HPV infection of the donors is known. The latter can only be reliably established by molecular means (Chapter 3) and may be critical since, for example, asymptomatic HPV 16-positive individuals may produce the most vigorous responses. Immunological studies should be extended to all patient groups, rather than only symptomatic patients, and in particular those that have recovered from disease.

Observations made so far with benign warts as a whole may be extrapolated to the high-risk HPVs, although one distinction must be stressed. Any extrapolations may only be relevant to HPV infection in the premalignant stages. The cancers should be regarded as a separate disease. While oncogenic HPVs are an essential component in the developmental pathway to malignancy, tumour cells may evade recognition by the immune system by variety of mechanisms not common to the benign tumours.

11.3   Immunogenicity of HPV

11.3.1   Evidence from cutaneous and mucosal warts

Much of the belief that high-risk HPV can be controlled by the immune system has been supported by observations of benign genital and cutaneous warts. Firstly, conditions of cellular immunosuppression are invariably associated with recrudescence of warts and a reduced incidence of spontaneous regression (reviewed by Benton *et al.* 1992). Generally, the incidence of warts, and of the occasional squamous carcinomas developing from the warts, increases with the duration of immunosuppression. Warts on immunosuppressed renal transplant patients often contain potentially oncogenic HPV types that are usually only seen in cases of epidermodysplasia verruciformis (Pfister *et al.* 1985). These types are likely to be responsible for the skin cancers seen.

Secondly, early studies of individuals with skin warts or condylomata suggest depressed cellular immunocompetence (Brodersen *et al.* 1974; Morison *et al.* 1975a, b, c; Chretien *et al.* 1978; Seski *et al.* 1978). Together these observations suggest that most of us are carriers of persistent or latent cutaneous HPV infections, which are normally adequately controlled by a healthy immune system. The chronic nature of many skin warts suggests that, in addition to reduced immunocompetence, warts may persist because of problems with accessibility or immunogenicity. Thirdly, benign warts regress. Some cutaneous warts can persist for several years, although approximately one third of typical skin warts resolve within six months (Bunney *et al.* 1992). The natural history of cervical lesions is not well documented, although an eight-year prospective study has shown that a quarter of all cervical lesions caused by HPV 6/11 regressed, a quarter progressed to higher-grade CIN, and the rest remained as persistent lesions (Syrjänen 1989). This is in contrast to lesions caused by the high-risk HPV types 16 and 18, which regressed in 5.6 per cent and 11.1 per cent of cases, respectively.

The stimuli for spontaneous regression are not known although there are striking histopathological similarities between regressing cutaneous warts and delayed type hypersensitivity (DTH) reactions, known to be mediated predominantly by T lymphocytes and macrophages (Tagami *et al.* 1985; Iwatsuki *et al.* 1986; Thivolet *et al.* 1982; Bender 1986; Berman and Winkelmann 1980). The observation that multiple cutaneous warts in disparate anatomical locations often resolve synchronously is also suggestive of a systemic immune response. This phenomenon can be induced by, for example, surgical ablation of selected genital warts, which often initiates the subsequent resolution of other untreated warts. Similarly, treatment with irritants such as podophylin, a topically applied plant extract that mediates its effects non-specifically by eliciting a localized inflammatory reaction, has a similar systemic effect. Together these observations suggest that viral antigens within a benign wart are normally inaccessible to antigen presenting cells, but are exposed upon mechanical disruption of the wart or during inflammatory infiltration.

There is thus good evidence for active involvement of the immune system (particularly cell-mediated immunity) in the protection against cutaneous HPV and resolution of the warts they cause. While this is encouraging for all HPVs, is there any similar evidence for protective responses against high-risk cervical infections? Although less numerous, there are reports of a higher incidence of high-grade CIN and cancers in immunosuppressed women (reviewed by Jablonska *et al.* 1989). On the other hand, rates of spontaneous regression of lesions containing HPV 16 or 18 is significantly lower than those containing 6 and 11 (Syrjänen, 1989), which implies a defect in immunological mechanisms. Instances where surgical ablation did not prevent the reappearance of additional lesions have been interpreted by some as evidence of reinfection of surrounding tissue, which may indicate that natural immunity to high-risk HPVs does not occur. Others have interpreted such observations as incomplete resection of infected tissue. Explanations remain contentious but do not preclude the existence of natural immunity against high risk HPVs.

11.3.2   Evidence from vaccines

As discussed in Chapter 10, vaccination of animals with a variety of crude, purified, or synthetic animal PV antigens can have both therapeutic and prophylactic properties against cutaneous papillomas. Prophylactic immunity against challenge with virus has been demonstrated in rabbits (Christensen *et al.* 1991; Lin *et al.* 1992) and in cattle (Pilacinski *et al.* 1984, 1986; Jin *et al.* 1989) and in each case protection is likely to be mediated by neutralizing antibodies. Therapeutic treatment of BPV-2 induced warts using recombinant BPV-2 L2 has also been demonstrated (Jarrett *et al.* 1991; Chapter 10) although it is not yet clear which cellular or humoral mechanisms are involved in regression.

The lack of a true animal model of CIN has had the effect of accelerating human vaccination trials. This is clearly the most direct means for determining the nature of protective responses, although the results of these trials will not be known for some time. Perhaps eliciting an HPV-specific response will be the least problematic aspect of any human vaccine; the delivery systems of such vaccines will be as critical as the choice of antigen (Crawford 1993). The only precedents for synthetic human vaccines consist of recombinant proteins adsorbed onto aluminium hydroxide (alum, which is currently the only adjuvant approved for human use) and administered intramuscularly. While many such vaccines have been produced and are undergoing trials, only one, the hepatitis B surface antigen produced in yeast (Ellis and Provost 1989) is approved. Such preparations produce high titres of specific antibody, and seem ideal for medium-term protection against pathogens accessible to antibody. However, extensive modifications in this regimen (particularly route of entry and formulation) will be necessary if mucosal IgA responses able to neutralize oncogenic HPVs is required. The development of recombinant bacterial and viral vectors for the induction of mucosal immunity to HPV 16 is being actively explored. These include the use of *Streptococcus* (Pozzi *et al.* 1992), *Lactobacilli* (Crawford *et al.* 1993), and poliovirus (Jenkins *et al.* 1990) as vectors. Alum-adsorbed preparations seem inadequate to elicit cytotoxic T cells, which may play a major role in the success of a therapeutic synthetic vaccine. This is likely to require live viral vectors such as recombinant vaccinia, or other means of producing the antigen within the cytoplasm of cells within the vaccinated host (see Chapter 8). Moreover, the route of immunization required to ensure homing of T cells to HPV-infected cells in the cervix are unknown.

11.3.3   Vaccines to cutaneous warts

How will vaccination against cutaneous warts assist in the design of vaccines against high-risk HPV? It is likely that the greatest area of influence will be in the design of immunotherapeutic strategies. Ultimately, the efficacy of therapeutic vaccines against high-risk cervical lesions will be difficult to assess, since it is unlikely that they could be administered in the absence of surgical treatment. At best, their role as an adjunct to surgery will be determined. In contrast there is generally no urgency to treat cutaneous warts, thus any vaccination strategy could be tested first without interference from other confounding therapies, and placebo controls (i.e., vector/adjuvant alone) could be performed without any ethical ramifications.

A second justification for developing vaccines to HPV 6/11 in particular is the recognition that the lesions caused by these viruses are significant problems in their own right. Most benign cutaneous and genital warts are generally perceived as no more than a nuisance, although they are a chronic problem for transplant patients who undergo life-long immunosuppression, and occasionally these skin and genital lesions become malignant. Genital warts often appear during immunosuppression, particularly during pregnancy, and current therapies consist mostly of surgical excision. These are unpleasant procedures and often ineffective, usually requiring repeated attempts. These lesions therefore represent an ideal system for testing novel immunotherapies. More importantly, transfer of genital wart HPVs during birth has been postulated to be the major mechanism of laryngeal infection of newborns. Laryngeal papillomas in infants are a more serious problem, requiring regular surgical removal to clear the airway.

11.4   Immunological basis of protective and other responses

The previous section outlined how studies of benign warts supported the view that HPVs are immunogenic. This has been postulated to differ between different HPV types, with the high-risk genital types being apparently less immunogenic than other types (Frazer and Tindle 1992). Comparative studies of immunity to the high and low-risk types will determine whether this is so and why. In this section I will examine the strategies that are being used to study natural responses to high-risk HPV in lieu of infectious particles, and how studies of cutaneous warts and their lesions have contributed to understanding HPV immunology.

11.4.1   Inflammatory reactions

The histological similarities between spontaneously regressing warts and typical inflammatory reactions have long been recognized, and topical application of irritants such as dinitrochlorobenzine or other mediators of local inflammation such as podophyllin have long been used as therapies for benign cutaneous warts (Bender 1985). Inflammation is a complex cascade of cellular and humoral elements, characterized by extravisation of leukocytes from local capillaries into the site. Inflammation can be triggered either by cutaneous phagocytes, or by antigen independent (non-specific) stimuli such as physical trauma. The phenotypes of the infiltrating cells differ, depending on the original stimulus and its persistence. Recently, CD4$^+$ and CD8$^+$ T lymphocytes have been identified infiltrating non-regressing (Viac *et al.* 1992) and regressing (Coleman *et al.* submitted for publication) benign warts by immunohistochemistry. Infiltration is accompanied by elevated expression of adhesion molecules, such as inter-cellular adhesion molecule 1 (ICAM-1), a ligand for the lymphocyte function related antigen 1 (LFA-1). Despite the wealth of histological data, the event(s) that initiates regression, and the mechanisms by which T cells eliminate infected cells, remain contentious. Mechanical or chemical disruption of the wart tissue to release viral antigens to surrounding antigen presenting cells may initiate regression is some cases, although this doesn't explain spontaneous regression. Elimination of infected cells may be by infiltrating cytotoxic leukocytes (see next section) or by the cytostatic/cytotoxic effects of soluble mediators liberated by infiltrating cells. The latter hypothesis has received some support from histochemical studies of spontaneously regressing Shope papillomas (Okabayashi *et al.* 1993), in which there appears to be a reduction in the proliferative activity of the tumour cells.

There seems little doubt that infiltrating T cells and antigen presenting cells play an important role in the resolution of benign warts, and the following observations suggest that a similar situation applies to HPV 16 infections. Priming of T cells to a particular antigen in the epithelium can often be demonstrated by a delayed-type hypersensitivity (DTH) response, an inflammatory reaction that normally develops 1–2 days after subsequent cutaneous challenge with the appropriate antigen. Accordingly, cutaneous administration of recombinant HPV 16 L1 protein in individuals that have CIN can elicit DTH reactions (Höpfl *et al.* 1991). Similarly, in an animal model in which natural epithelial HPV infection is simulated by grafting HPV 16 E7-transfected murine keratinocytes onto syngeneic mice, subsequent intradermal challenge with recombinant vaccinia virus expressing HPV 16 E7 induces DTH that is both antigen-specific and CD4$^+$ T lymphocyte-dependent (McLean *et al.* 1992). Together these observations argue very strongly that certain HPV 16 antigens can be recognized by the skin associated lymphoid tissue and elicit a T cell response. Like other cutaneous skin tests (particularly the Mantoux test for *Mycobacterium tuberculosis* immunity), they may allow us to monitor current immunity to HPV. A similar cutaneous test may be used to reveal cytotoxic T cell priming *in vivo* (Kündig *et al.* 1992). Such tests represent both useful diagnostic tools in the quest to correlate immune responsiveness with disease status, in addition to representing important effector mechanism in the resolution of warts.

As is the case for cutaneous warts, induction of inflammation may also be of value for the therapy of high-grade CIN. However, problems in evaluating the efficacy are the same as discussed above for vaccines. Thus these, along with a battery of other potential molecular and chemotherapeutic strategies, are likely only to be used as an adjunct to surgery.

11.4.2   Cytotoxic T cells

Cell mediated cytotoxicity is a phenomenon mediated by a variety of different leucocytes, including $CD4^+$ and $CD8^+$ lymphocytes, lymphokine-activated killer (LAK) cells, and natural killer (NK) cells. Our understanding of the molecular basis of recognition by these effector cells differs between extremes. Each has different requirements for stimulation resulting in each having a specialized role within a complementary arsenal directed against cells in the body that have become altered by viral or neoplastic transformation. Much of the discussion below is focused on classical cytotoxic $CD8^+$ T lymphocytes. This is reflective only of the wealth of molecular detail we have concerning T cell recognition and the demonstrable importance of CTL in the other model virus or tumour systems. The importance of CTL in HPV infection, whether occurring naturally or induced by vaccination, is presently unknown but is under intensive research. The attraction is that our extensive understanding of how these cells recognize antigen allows us to design the vaccines rationally.

The molecular basis of T cell recognition is discussed in detail in Chapters 8 and 9. Central to this recognition are nascent heterodimeric HLA molecules (for human leukocyte antigen), encoded by genes in the major histocompatibility complex (MHC) which, during transport to the cell surface, complex with peptides produced by the enzymatic degradation of self and foreign proteins and display them at the cell surface to the antigen receptors of T cells. HLA molecules are classified into class I and class II, based on their structure, locus within the MHC, and phenotype of the corresponding acceptor T cell. The ligand for the antigen receptors of $CD8^+$ CTL are peptides presented by class I HLA molecules. Most viral infections elicit responses from CTL, which in turn play a significant part in the elimination of the virus by killing infected cells. Strategies employed by different viruses to evade recognition by CTL (Browne *et al.* 1990; Pircher *et al.* 1990; Burgert and Kvist 1985; Del Val *et al.* 1988; Phillips *et al.* 1991) provide indirect evidence of their importance. However, the real impetus for wishing to detect and generate HPV-specific CTL comes from findings in many viral systems that CTL, elicited *in vivo* by synthetic antigenic preparations, including recombinant viral vectors (Klavinskis *et al.* 1989; Sumner *et al.* 1991) or by peptides mimicking the CTL epitope (Kast *et al.* 1991) can confer protection to animals from subsequent challenge with the virus. The implications of these animal studies for immunotherapy of HPV in humans are exciting. Natural HPV-specific CTL responses could be boosted, or induced by vaccination where no response existed before.

A critical prerequisite, however, for recognition by CTL is transport and display of processed HPV peptides by class I MHC molecules on the surface of HPV-infected keratinocytes. Thus if HPV employs evasive strategies any induced CTL responses will be less effective. Encouraging animal studies, some discussed below, have shown that CTL can kill targets expressing HPV 16 L1, E6, and E7 proteins. Provided these responses are shown to be HPV specific, they indicate that there is nothing inherent about these antigens that prevents their processing into peptide epitopes and presentation to CTL at the surface of the infected cell. However, in these studies the HPV proteins are expressed artificially (by DNA mediated gene transfer or viral vectors), usually out of context of the whole HPV genome, and in cells other than human cervical keratinocytes. Thus, at present it is unknown whether premalignant or malignant cervical keratinocytes are a suitable target for CTL. A direct approach to address whether HPV antigens are accessible to CTL is by the elution of naturally processed peptides from class I molecules affinity purified from HPV infected keratinocytes, followed by sequencing to identify their source (Van Bleek and Nathenson, 1990; Hill *et al.* 1992). This is technically difficult: large numbers of cells are required and successful sequencing depends on the relative abundance of the peptide.

CTL to HPV 16

Naturally occurring CTL responses to HPV in humans have been notoriously difficult to demonstrate. The conventional approach, as applied to other viruses such as influenza virus and EBV, is to use the virus to infect their natural host cell and use these to stimulate CTL within autologous bulk populations of peripheral blood mononuclear cells (PBMC) *in vitro*. The CTL are then detected in ^{51}Cr release assays using autologous target cells (usually lymphoblastoid cell lines) infected with the virus. By using target cells infected with recombinant vaccinia virus recombinants expressing individual genes from the parent virus, it is possible to identify the viral antigen(s) the CTL recognize. The epitopes can be precisely mapped using synthetic peptides that mimic the naturally processed peptide epitopes expressed at the surface of the infected cell, and the use of targets matched at single HLA loci with the donor enables the restricting HLA molecules to be identified. This stands in contrast to HPV 16, where the absence of infectious virus has made necessary the production of alternative sources of antigen for the propagation and assay of HPV-specific CTL.

Given these considerations, CTL studies are being approached from different directions. One is to generate CTL responses in animals. This enables us to learn more about the immunogenicity of HPV antigens and to evaluate their potential for eliciting effective anti-tumour responses. To elicit CTL, animals are vaccinated with syngeneic cells transfected with HPV 16 DNA, or HPV/vaccinia recombinants, or synthetic peptides representing naturally processed HPV-derived epitopes. As a readout, the induction of HPV 16 specific CTL, or the retardation of HPV 16 expressing tumour cells, are most widely used. For example, a significant percentage of rats vaccinated and boosted intradermally with vaccinia recombinants expressing E6 or E7 (but not E5) show retarded or arrested tumour development after challenge 16 days later with tumourigenic fibroblasts cotransfected with complete HPV 16 and c-Ha-*ras* (Meneguzzi *et al.* 1991). Since the only common antigens expressed by the recombinant vaccinia and the transfected fibroblasts is E6 or E7, the protective immune response is likely to be directed against these antigens, or a cellular protein induced by them. Similarly, mice are protected from syngeneic HPV 16 E7-expressing melanoma cells by coimmunization with non-tumourigenic fibroblasts that also express transfected E7 (Chen *et al.* 1991). Similar results were obtained with HPV 16 E6 (Chen *et al.* 1992). Although the mechanism for protection is not known in these animal models, the 'vaccines' used (vaccinia-HPV recombinants and HPV-expressing transfected cells) should elicit protective HPV-specific CTL. Further evidence for CTL involvement comes from *in vivo* administration of anti-CD8 antibody that blocked protection (Chen *et al.* 1991), and the ability to isolate CD8$^+$ CTL from protected mice (Chen *et al.* 1992). Firmer evidence that murine or human responses are HPV-specific will come from the use of synthetic peptides representing HPV epitopes to pulse target cells in CTL assays. This also allows epitopes recognized by CTL to be mapped, the MHC restriction of the epitopes to be identified, and the direct testing of these epitopes as a peptide vaccine.

Until equivalent experiments in humans (i.e., vaccine trials) are underway, a number of different approaches are used to study human HPV-specific CTL. One is to identify putative CTL epitopes on the basis of binding to class I HLA molecules. Two routes can be taken; the longer is to screen individual synthetic peptides spanning the antigenic sequence for binding to particular HLA molecules. Synthetic peptides spanning the antigen are screened for their ability to bind to or stabilize class I MHC alleles on the mutant murine and human cell lines RMA-S (which expresses H-2 K^b and D^b) and .174/T2 (which expresses HLA A2.1), respectively. Both cells have an increased capacity to bind extracellular peptide, a property that has been exploited as a peptide-MHC binding assay (Townsend *et al.* 1989; Stauss *et al.* 1992; Elvin *et al.* 1993). The short-cut approach is predict putative CTL epitopes on the basis of possession of an allele-specific anchor motif (Falk *et al.* 1991; Jardetzky *et al.* 1991; Hill *et al.* 1992; DiBrino *et al.* 1993; Suhrbier *et al.* 1993; Sutton *et al.* 1993). These approaches are particularly attractive for HPV CTL epitope mapping because they are independent of pre-existing CTL. However, their relevance must eventually be demonstrated by showing that the CTL elicited to them recognize targets expressing the naturally processed epitopes (i.e., targets expressing the whole antigen intracellularly). Many studies indicate that most dominant CTL epitopes mapped by conventional means, turn out to be strong binders to MHC class I and/or contain motifs (Townsend *et al.* 1986; Gotch *et al.* 1987; Falk *et al.* 1991; Morrison *et al.* 1992; Elvin *et al.* 1993), and other, longer peptide epitopes have been optimized using motifs (Carbone and Bevan 1989; Rötzschke *et al.* 1991; Lipford *et al.* 1993; Sutton *et al.* 1993). There are likely to be exceptions to this simplistic view. Nevertheless, motifs and binding data are being used successfully to predict novel immunodominant CTL epitopes (Palmer *et al.* 1991; Hill *et al.* 1992; Lipford *et al.* 1993; Suhrbier *et al.* 1993; Elvin *et al.* 1993).

HPV 16 E6 and E7 seem to be examples where these simple predictive rules do not hold, at least in the context of the mouse immune system. While there is a good correlation between peptides of E6 and E7 binding to K^b and D^b and their ability to elicit CTL, these peptides are not the ones recognized by CTL elicited to naturally processed peptides. Even the possession of an allele-specific anchor motif does not ensure recognition by these CTL (see Chapter 8). As such, they may represent subdominant or silent epitopes, which although satisfying the dual requirements of MHC binding and T cell receptor recognition, are nevertheless not the products of natural processing of the viral antigen by murine cells. Whether this finding holds for HPV 16 antigens processed by human cells remains to be determined.

CTL to cutaneous HPV

This is a largely unexplored area. To address this we have used the HLA A2.1 motif described by Falk *et al.* (1991) to locate putative CTL epitopes in HPV 6b and 11. Three nonapeptides from the E7 ORFs were tested for their ability to stimulate CTL. When presented by autologous antigen presenting cells, all three stimulate peptide-specific, A2-restricted CTL from donors with and without overt genital warts. Moreover, CTL to peptide HPV11E7 4–12 kill targets infected with recombinant vaccinia expressing the whole protein. In reciprocal experiments, CTL stimulated *in vitro* with antigen presenting cells infected with vaccinia expressing whole E7 killed targets pulsed with the 4–12 peptide (Tarpey *et al.* 1994). Thus for one peptide at least, the motif provided a convenient short-cut. The protocol used (based on that described by Macatonia *et al.* 1991) was intended to prime *in vitro*, but studies are underway to determine whether this is the case or whether we are stimulating a memory pool of CTL, and whether the methodologies using this peptide or the vaccinia recombinants are useful reagents for detecting naturally occurring CTL.

11.4.3   Helper T cells and lymphoproliferation assay

Helper T cells are a heterogeneous population of T cells that function *in vivo* to produce cytokines required for the differentiation of B lymphocytes and CTL into effector cells. The term 'helper T cells', however, is used synonymously with T cells that are detected by antigen-specific proliferation *in vitro*. In reality, the population of proliferative T cells only partially overlaps with helper T cells. A number of lymphoproliferation studies have been performed, both in humans and in animal models, but little is known about cytokine responses to HPV.

Most human proliferative studies have been performed using polyclonal T cell lines obtained from peripheral blood and stimulated *in vitro* with recombinant protein. In cases where virions are available, these have also been used as antigen (see below). In animal models, responder T cells are primed by immunization with protein emulsified in adjuvant. By using whole antigen in these ways the T cells that respond to naturally processed epitopes are stimulated. These T cells can then be tested for proliferative responses using individual synthetic peptides spanning the antigen to map the immunodominant regions. It is important to recognise that, as with CTL, there are also likely to be subdominant or silent epitopes, which although as synthetic peptides may bind to class II MHC molecules and be recognized by T cells, may not be the products of natural processing.

As described in the introduction, the rationale for detecting HPV-specific helper T cells is the same as for cytotoxicity or for antibodies: evidence of natural response; correlation with disease and identification of responses associated with protection; and determine efficacy of vaccines. In addition, helper T cell epitope mapping has particular significance in the design of multivalent (synthetic peptide-based) vaccines since the inclusion of helper epitopes is important for induction of antibodies and possibly cytotoxic T cells, and to prime the host for a T-cell memory response (see review by Zanetti *et al.* 1987). The importance of the conformation of the HPV test antigen is usually assumed not to be relevant owing to its processing into peptides by the antigen presenting cell (APC) prior to presentation to T cells. For this reason, synthetic proteins and peptides should provide ideal reagents to explore this immunological aspect of the high-risk HPVs. It must be emphasized that *in vivo*, however, native virus would be expected to be processed by different clones of B cells (by virtue of antigen receptor-mediated uptake) than non-native antigen, thereby resulting in the production of polyclonal sera with different binding specificities.

High-risk HPV

In animal models, helper T cells that have been primed *in vivo* using fusion proteins have been assayed in *in vitro* proliferation assays against synthetic peptides. By using such methods immunodominant regions, presented by various murine class II alleles, have been mapped in HPV 16 E7 (Tindle *et al*. 1991; Commerford *et al*. 1991; Shepherd *et al*. 1992). Lymphoproliferative responses in humans have been more difficult to interpret owing to the previous history of HPV infection of the donors being largely unknown. Positive but small lymphoproliferative responses have been observed in CIN patients to HPV 16 and 18 E6 fusion proteins, but not to E4 (Cubie *et al*. 1989). More recently, Shepherd and colleagues have found that T cells from patients with cervical cancer proliferate to HPV 16 L1 fusion protein *in vitro* and have localized this to epitopes within the region 305–345 (personal communication).

Before fusion proteins were widely available, Strang *et al*. (1990) used predictive methods to identify four putative human epitopes in HPV 16 L1 in one in E6. Proliferating T cell lines and clones were established from two asymptomatic laboratory personnel; the authors suggested that these responses were due to priming of the T cells by natural infection and that subclinical HPV 16 infection can exist in the 'normal' population. However, it was not demonstrated whether these T cells recognized naturally processed antigen. Until proven otherwise, these epitopes may be subdominant and were detected owing to *in vitro* T cell priming.

Cutaneous HPV

The areas in which cutaneous wart HPVs offer unique opportunities for lymphoproliferative studies are two-fold. One is the facility with which responses can be correlated with regression. The second is the use of native virions for use as antigen for stimulating T cells *in vitro*. Early studies with pooled skin wart extracts and purified virus particles as antigen (Lee and Eisinger 1976; Ivanyi and Morison *et al*. 1976) demonstrated that low levels of lymphoproliferation were detected in people with or without prior histories of skin warts. Responses seemed lowest in individuals with more persistent warts. However, these pioneering studies are difficult to interpret since they were performed before the heterogeneity of HPV genotypes was known and molecular genotyping technology widely available. More recent experiments with purified HPV-1 and 2 particles (Charleson *et al*. 1992) also revealed that the magnitude and prevalence of proliferative responses by donors with HPV 1 or 2 infection are low. This is in spite of these individuals having otherwise normal proliferative responses to HSV (in patients with a clinical history of herpes) or to mitogen. Moreover, there was no obvious correlation between responsiveness and clinical status of the wart.

There is insufficient data so far to draw any meaningful conclusions regarding the importance of the T cells detected in proliferation assay in the control of HPV infection. The difference in magnitude of proliferative responses seen by different groups indicates that these assays are influenced by many factors in addition to whether T cells have been primed to antigen *in vivo*. These could include patient group (HLA type, T cell repertoire, and immunocompetence), status of HPV lesion, HPV status of control donors, quality and quantity of test antigen, T cell responder frequency in samples taken, and assay conditions.

11.4.4   T cells: Naturally occurring or primed *in vitro*?

Under appropriate but ill-defined conditions, primary cytotoxic and proliferative T cell responses can be elicited *in vitro* from naive T cells (Sambhara *et al*. 1990; Macatonia *et al*. 1991). It is thought that professional antigen presenting cells, particularly dendritic cells and activated B cells, are the only cells able to prime by virtue of providing essential costimulatory signals, such as the B7 molecule (Schwartz 1992), in conjunction with processed antigenic peptides. Where the aim has been to identify epitopes rather than to define naturally occurring T cells, *in vitro* priming can be an advantage. However, in experiments aimed at detecting naturally occurring T cell responses induced after infection or vaccination, it will be important to distinguish whether detected responses are an artefact. For this reason, stimulation of proliferative and cytotoxic T cells with naturally processed whole protein may be preferable over synthetic peptides.

11.4.5   Antibodies

Serological studies of HPV have many important applications. Firstly, the ability to detect specifically responses to high-risk genital HPV may be used to correlate responses with the presence or absence of disease, or possibly with different stages of disease. This may provide the clinician with useful prognosticative information. Secondly, seroepidemiological studies may aid conventional (molecular) detection systems to resolve the issues concerning prevalence of disease, how high-risk HPVs are transmitted, other factors associated with resistance and susceptibility, and the efficacy of prophylactic vaccination. Thirdly, an understanding of antibody neutralization of HPV may improve vaccine design, help identify the HPV receptor, or allow the HPVs to be classified according to serotypes rather than the present system. In the absence of native particles, researchers have resorted to a number of synthetic antigens (see review by Galloway and Jenison 1990). There is much debate over the relative merits of recombinant proteins verses synthetic peptides, and denaturing detection systems (Western blotting) verses non-denaturing (ELISA, immunoprecipitation, *in vitro* transcription-translation).

Cutaneous HPV

The main impact that human cutaneous warts have had in this field is the availability of virions. This stands in contrast to virions of high-risk genital HPV, which are noticeably absent from cervical biopsy material. This has been hypothesized (M. A. Stanley, personal communication) to be due to the constant exofoliation of the cervical mucosa. In a key study, Steele and Gallimore (1990) exploited the availability of HPV1 particles from plantar warts to directly compare the effect of particle denaturation on their ability to be immunoprecipitated by human sera. The majority of the sera were only able to detect native particles, indicating that, for HPV1 at least, the response is directed largely against conformational epitopes. Studies with HPV 11 particles produced in the xenograft system indicate that HPV 11 neutralization epitopes are also conformational. In these studies, rabbit antisera to HPV 11, BPV 1, or CRPV neutralized the original virus used to immunize but not the other two viruses (Christensen and Kreider 1990). Moreover, human sera that reacted in ELISA with native HPV 11 neutralized infectivity of HPV 11, whereas sera that only recognized denatured HPV 11 did not neutralize (Christensen *et al*. 1992). Immunoelectron microscopy has also been used to detect antibodies in serum (Anisimová *et al*. 1990) but this would seem a rather cumbersome technique for routine use.

While such studies have raised speculation about the interpretation of 'non-native antigen' serology, none of the studies using native particles preclude the use of non-native antigens either for specifically detecting naturally occurring antibodies, or for eliciting neutralizing antibodies as a vaccine. For example, epitopes common to many papillomaviruses exposed by virion denaturation are detected particularly well by sera from patients with genital warts (Christensen 1992). Animal vaccination studies (see Chapter 10) indicate that non-native recombinant capsid proteins provide good protection against warts in subsequent challenge with virus. Moreover, there are a growing number of examples where non-native antigens do discriminate between responses during different disease states (Christensen *et al*. 1992). Much of the speculation hinges on comparing both types of antigens in serological assays to determine the strengths and limitations to be expected. As this validation of synthetic reagents has become a major exercise for many laboratories, the contribution played by native cutaneous HPV will continue to be a significant one.

Synthetic virus-like particles have been made of HPV 1 (Hagensee *et al*. 1993), HPV 11 (Rose *et al*. 1993), HPV 16 (Zhou *et al*. 1991; Kirnbauer *et al*. 1992), and BPV1 (Kirnbauer *et al*. 1992; Zhou *et al*. 1993) but even these will need to be compared with the genuine article. For benign wart

HPVs this is possible, and the early signs are very encouraging. Purified BPV 1 L1 particles can elicit very high titres of rabbit antibodies able to neutralize native BPV- 1 in the focus-inhibition assay, whereas antisera to disrupted particles fail to neutralize (Kirnbauer *et al.* 1992). Similarly, non-denatured cell lysates containing HPV 11 L1 particles detect reactivity in rabbit antisera to native virions, and in human sera shown previously to react with native virions, whereas reactivity by these sera is lost when the lysates are denatured (Rose *et al.* 1993). These studies reflect the findings seen when native virions are used as the detection antigen, and strongly suggest that synthetic particles may be reliably used in their place.

11.5   Conclusions

The clinical significance of cutaneous warts is often overshadowed by the oncogenic or high-risk genital HPV types. It is they that are perceived as producing the more serious clinical problem and it is they that are the focus of immunological research and vaccine design. High-risk HPVs are particularly difficult viruses to understand at the immunological level and much of what we believe about them has been extrapolated from the study of cutaneous warts. There is little doubt that cutaneous warts provide unique opportunities for immunological study. In particular, the immuno- logical basis of regression, the availability of native virions, and especially in the development of novel immunotherapeutic strategies. Their true importance is thus seen in terms of how they further our understanding of the high-risk HPVs. In addition, benign cutaneous and mucosal warts are significant problems in their own right and afflict many more people than cervical cancer.

Acknowledgements

The author would like to thank Philip Shepherd for sharing unpublished data, and Robert Tindle, Philip Shepherd, Julian Hickling, Hans Stauss, Simon Stacey, and Ian Tarpey for their insights. The HPV 6/11 CTL experiments discussed were supported by the Cancer Research Campaign.

References

Anisomová, E., Bartak, P. Vlcek, D. Hirsch, I. Brichacek, B., and Vonka, V. (1990). *Journal of General Virology*, **71**, 419–22.
Bender, M. E. (1986). Concepts of wart regression. *Archives of Dermatology*, **122**, 644–7.

Benton, C., Shahdullah, H., and Hunter, J. A. A. (1992). Human papillomavirus in the immunocompromised. *Papillomavirus Report*, **3**, 23–6.

Berman, A. and Winkelmann, R. K. (1980). Involuting common warts. Clinical and histopathologic findings. *Journal of American Academy of Dermatology*, **3**, 356–62.

Brodersen, I., Genner, J., and Brodthagen, H. (1974). Tuberculin sensitivity in BCG-vaccinated children with common warts. *Acta Dermato-venerelogica*, **54**, 291–2.

Browne, H., Smith G., Beck, S., and Minson, T. (1990). A complex between the MHC class I homologue encoded by human cytomegalovirus and β_2 microglobulin. *Nature*, **347**, 770–2.

Bunney, M. H., Benton, E. C., and Cubie, H. A. (1992). *Viral warts: biology and treatments*, 2nd edn. Oxford University Press, Oxford.

Burgert, H-G. and Kvist, S. (1985). An adenovirus type 2 glycoprotein blocks cell surface expression of human histocompatibility class I antigens. *Cell*, **41**, 987–97.

Carbone, F. R. and Bevan, M. J. (1989). Induction of ovalbumin-specific cytotoxic T cells by *in vivo* peptide immunization. *Journal of Experimental Medicine*, **169**, 603–12.

Chen, L., Kinney Thomas, E., Hu, S-L, Hellström, I., and Hellström, K. E. (1991). Human papillomavirus type 16 nucleoprotein E7 is a tumour rejection antigen. *Proceedings of the National Academy of Sciences (USA)*, **88**, 110–14.

Chen, L., Mizuno, M. T., Singhal, M. C., Hu, S.-L., Galloway, D. A., Hellström, I., and Hellström, K. E. (1992). Induction of cytotxic T lymphocytes specific for a syngeneic tumor expressing the E6 oncoprotein of human papillomavirus type 16. *Journal of Immunology*, **148**, 2617–21.

Chretien, J. H., Esswein, J. G., and Garagusi, V. F. (1978). Decreased T cell levels in patients with warts. *Archives of Dermatology*, **114**, 213–15.

Charleson, F. C., Norval, M., Benton, E. C., and Hunter, J. A. A. (1992). Lymphoproliferative responses to human papillomaviruses in patients with cutaneous warts. *British Journal of Dermatology*, **127**, 551–9.

Christensen, N. D. and Kreider, J. W. (1990). Antibody mediated neutralization *in vivo* of infectious papillomaviruses. *Journal of Virology*, **64**, 3151–6.

Christensen, N. D., Kreider, J. W., Kan, N. C., and DiAngelo, S. L. (1991). The open reading frame L2 of cottontail rabbit papillomavirus contains antibody-neutralizing epitopes. *Virology*, **181**, 572–9.

Christensen, N. D., Kreider, J. W., Shah, K. V., and Rando, R. F. (1992). Detection of human serum antibodies that neutralize infectious human papillomavirus type 11 virions. *Journal of General Virology*, **73**, 1261–7.

Commerford, S. A., McCance, D. J., Dougan, G., and Tite, J. P. (1991). Identification of T- and B-cell epitopes of the E7 protein of human papillomavirus type 16. *Journal of Virology*, **65**, 4681–90.

Crawford, L. (1993). Prospects for cervical cancer vaccines. In *The molecular pathology of cancer* (eds. N. R. Lamoins and N. A. Wright). Cancer Surveys Vol. 16, pp. 215–29. Cold Spring Laboratory Press.

Cubie, H. A., Norval, M., Crawford, L., Banks, L., and Crook, T. (1989). Lymphoproliferative response to fusion proteins of human papillomaviruses in patients with cervical neoplasia. *Epidemiology & Infection*, **103**, 625–32.

Del Val, M., Münch, K., Reddehase, M. J., and Koszinowski, U. H. (1989).

Presentation of CMV immediate-early antigen to cytolytic T lymphocytes is selectively prevented by viral genes expressed in the early phase. *Cell*, **58**, 305–15.

DiBrino, M., Parker, K. C., Shiloach, J., Knierman, M., Lukszo, J., Turner, R. V., *et al.* (1993). Endogenous peptides bound to HLA-A3 possess a specific combination of anchor residues that permit identification of potential antigenic epitopes. *Proceedings of the National Academy of Sciences (USA)*, **90**, 1508–12.

Ellis, R. W. and Provost, P. J. (1989). Hepatitis B and A vaccines. In *Recent developments in prophylactic immunization* (ed. A. J. Zuckerman), pp. 181–209. Kluwer Academic Publishers, London.

Elvin, J., Potter, C., Elliot, T., Cerundolo, and Townsend, A. (1993) A method to quantify binding of unlabelled peptides to class I MHC molecules and detect their allele specificity. *Journal of Immunological Methods*, **158**, 161–71.

Falk, K., Rötzschke, O., Stevanović, S., Jung, G., and Rammensee, H-G. 1991. Allele-specific motifs revealed by sequencing of self-peptides eluted from MHC molecules. *Nature*, **351**, 290–6.

Frazer, I. H. and Tindle, R. W. (1992). Cell-mediated immunity to papillomaviruses. *Papillomavirus Report*, **3**, 53–8.

Galloway, D. A. and Jenison, S. A. (1990). Characterization of the humoral immune response to genital papillomaviruses. *Molecular & Biological Medicine*, **7**, 59–72.

Gotch, F., Rothbard, J. B., Howland, K., Townsend, A., and McMichael, A. (1987). Cytotoxic T lymphocytes recognize a fragment of influenza virus matrix protein in association with HLA-A2. *Nature*, **326**, 881–2.

Hagensee, M. E., Yaegashi, N., and Galloway, D. A. (1993). Self-assembly of human papillomavirus type 1 capsids by expression of the L1 protein alone or by coexpression of the L1 and L2 capsid proteins. *Journal of Virology*, **67**, 315–22.

Hill, A. V. S., Elvin, J., Willis, A. C., Aidoo, M., Allsopp, C. E. M., Gotch, F. M., *et al.* (1992). Molecular analysis of the association of HLA-B53 and resistance to severe malaria. *Nature*, **360**, 434–9.

Höpfl, R., Sandbichler, M., Sepp, N., Heim, K., Müller-Holzner, E., Wartsuch B., *et al.* (1991). Skin test for HPV type 16 proteins in cervical intra-epithelial neoplasia. *The Lancet*, **337**, 373–4.

Ivanyi, L. and Morison, W. L. (1976). *In vitro* lymphocyte stimulation by wart antigens in man. *British Journal of Dermatology*, **94**, 523–7.

Iwatsuki, K., Tagami M., Takigawa, M., and Yamada, M. (1986). Plane warts under spontaneous regression. Immunopathologic study on cellular constituents leading to the inflammatory reaction. *Archives of Dermatology*, **122**, 655–9.

Jablonska, S., Majewski, S., and Malejczyk, J. (1989). HPV infection and immunological responses. In *Genitoanal papilloma virus infection* (eds. G. von Krogh and E. Rylander) Chapter X, pp. 289–329. Conpharm AB, Karlstad.

Jardetzky, T. S., Lane, W. S., Robinson, R. A., Madden, D. R., and Wiley, D. C. (1991). Identification of self peptides bound to purified HLA-B27. *Nature*, **353**, 326–9.

Jarrett, W. F. J., Smith, K. T., O'Neil, B. W., Gaukroger, J. M., Chandrachud, L. M., Grindlay, G. J., *et al.* (1991). Studies on vacciniation against papillomaviruses: prophylactic and therapeutic vaccination with recombinant structural proteins. *Virology*, **184**, 33–42.

Jenkins, O., Cason, J., Burke, K. L., Lunney, D., Gillen, A., Patel, D., *et al.* (1990). An antigen chimera of poliovirus induces antibodies against human papillomavirus type 16. *Journal of Virology*, **64**, 1201–6.

Jin, X. W., Cowsert, L. M., Pilacinski, W. P. and Jenson, A. B, (1989). Identification of L2 open reading frame products of bovine papillomavirus type 1 using monoclonal antibodies. *Journal of General Virology*, **70**, 1133–40.

Kast, W. M., Roux, L., Curren, J., Blom, H. J. J., Voordouw, A. C., Meloen, R. H., *et al.* (1991). Protection against lethal sendai virus infection by *in vivo* priming of virus-specific cytotoxic T lymphocytes with a free synthetic peptide. *Proceedings of the National Academy of Sciences (USA)*, **88**, 2238–47.

Kirnbauer, R., Booy, F., Cheng, N., Lowy, D. R., and Schiller, J. T. (1992). Papillomavirus L1 major capsid protein self-assembles into virus-like particles that are highly immunogenic. *Proceedings of the National Academy of Sciences (USA)*, **89**, 12180–4.

Klavinskis, L. S., Whitton, J. L., and Oldstone, M. B. A. (1989). Molecularly engineered vaccine which expresses an immunodominant T-cell epitope induces cytotoxic T lymphocytes that confer protection from lethal virus infection. *Journal of Virology*, **63**, 4311–16.

Kündig, T. M., Althage, A., Hengartner, H., and Zinkernagel, R. M. (1992). Skin test to assess virus-specific cytotoxic T-cell activity. *Proceedings of the National Academy of Sciences (USA)*, **89**, 7757–61.

Lee, A. K. Y. and Eisinger, M. (1976). Cell-mediated immunity (CMI) to human wart virus and wart-associated tissue antigens. *Clinical & Experimental Immunology*, **26**, 419–24.

Lin, Y.-L., Borenstein, L. A., Selvakumar, R., Ahmed, R., and Wettstein, F. O. (1992). Effective vaccination against papilloma development by immunization with L1 or L2 structural protein of cottontail rabbit papillomavirus. *Virology*, **66**, 1655–64.

Lipford, G. B., Hoffman, M., Wagner, H., and Heeg, K. (1993). Primary *in vivo* responses to ovalbumin. Probing the predictive value of the Kb binding motif. *Journal of Immunology*, **150**, 1212–22.

Macatonia, S. E., Patterson, S. and Knight, S. C. (1991) Primary proliferative and cytotoxic T-cell responses to HIV induced *in vitro* by human dendritic cells. *Immunology*, **74**, 399–406.

McLean, C. S., Sterling, J. S., Mowat, J., Nash, A. A., and Stanley, M. A. (1993). Delayed-type hypersensitivity response to the human papillomavirus type 16 E7 protein in a mouse model. *Journal of General Virology*, **74**, 239–45.

Meneguzzi, G. Cerni, C. Kieny, M. P., and Lathe, R. (1991). Immunization against human papillomavirus type 16 tumour cells with recombinant vaccinia viruses expressing E6 and E7. *Virology*, **181**, 62–9.

Meyers, C., Frattini, M. G., Hudson, J. B., and Laimins, L. A. (1992). Biosynthesis of human papillomavirus from a continuous cell line upon epithelial differentiation. *Science*, **257**, 971–3.

Morison, W. L. (1975a). Viral warts, herpes simplex and herpes zoster in patients with secondary immune deficiencies and neoplasms. *British Journal of Dermatology*, **92**, 625–30.

Morison, W. L. (1975b). *In vitro* assay of immunity to human wart antigen. *British Journal of Dermatology*, **93**, 545–52.

Morison, W. L. (1975c). Cell-mediated immune responses in patients with warts. *British Journal of Dermatology*, **93**, 553–6.

Morrison, J., Elvin, J., Latron, F., Gotch, F., Moots, R., Strominger, J., and McMichael, A. (1992). Identification of the nonomer peptide from influenza A matrix protein and the role of pockets of HLA-A2 in its recognition by cytotoxic T lymphocytes. *European Journal of Immunology*, **22**, 903–7.

Obalek, S., Glinski, W., Haftek, M. *et al.* (1980). Comparative studies on cell-mediated immunity in patients with different warts. *Dermatologica*, **161**, 73–83.

Okabayashi, M., Angell, M. G., Budgeon, L. R., and Kreider, J. W. (1993). Shope papilloma cell and leukocyte proliferation in regressing and progressing lesions. *American Journal of Pathology*, **142**, 489–6.

Palmer, E. G., Harty, J. T., and Bevan, M. J. (1991). Precise prediction of a dominant class I MHC-restricted epitope of *Lysteria monocytogenes*. *Nature*, **353**, 852–5.

Pfister H., Iftner, T. and Fuchs, P. G. (1985). Papillomaviruses from epidermodysplasia verruciformis patients and renal allograft recipients. In *Papillomaviruses: molecular and clinical aspects*, (eds. P. M. Howley and T. R. Broker), pp. 85–100. Liss, New York.

Phillips, R. E., Rowland-Jones, S., Nixon, D. F., Gotch, F. M., Edwards, J. P., Ogunlesi, A. O., *et al.* (1991). Human immunodeficiency virus genetic variation that can escape cytotoxic T cell recognition. *Nature*, **354**, 453–9.

Pilacinski, W. P., Glassman, D. L., Krzyzek, R. A., Sadowski, P. L., and Robbins, A. K. (1984). Cloning and expression in *Escherichia coli* of the bovine papillomavirus L1 and L2 open reading frames. *BioTechnology*, **2**, 356–60.

Pilacinski, W. P., Glassman, D. L., Glassman, K. F., Reed, D. E., Lum, M. A., *et al.* (1986). Immunization against bovine papillomavirus infection. In *Papillomaviruses* (Ciba Foundation Symposium 120), pp. 136–56. Wiley, Chichester.

Pircher, H., Moskophidis, D., Rohrer, U., Bürki, K., Hengartner, H., and Zinkernagel, R. M. (1990). Viral escape by selection of cytotoxic T cell-resistant virus variants *in vivo*. *Nature*, **346**, 629–32.

Pozzi, G., Contorni, M., Oggioni, M. R., Manganelli, R., Tommasino, M., Cavalieri, F. *et al.* (1992). Delivery and expression of a heterologous antigen on the surface of streptococci. *Infection & Immunity*, **60**, 1902–7.

Rose R. C., Bonnez, W., Reichman, R. C., and Garcea, R. L. (1993). Expression of human papillomavirus type 11 L1 protein in insect cells: in vivo and in vitro assembly of viruslike particles. *Journal of Virology*, **67**, 1936–44.

Rötzschke, O., Falk, K., Stevanovic, S., Jung, G., Walden, P., and Rammensee, H.-G. (1991). Exact prediction of a natural T cell epitope. *European Journal of Immunology*, **21**, 2891–4.

Sambhara, S. R., Upadhya, A. G., and Miller, R. G. (1990). Generation and characterization of peptide-specific, MHC-restricted cytotoxic T lymphocyte (CTL) and helper T cell lines from unprimed T cells under microculture conditions. *Journal of Immunological Methods*, **130**, 101–9.

Schwartz, R. H. (1992). Costimulation of T lymphocytes: the role of CD28, CTLA-4, and B7/BB1 in interleukin-2 production and immunotherapy. *Cell*, **71**, 1065–8.

Seski, J. C., Reinhalter, E. R., and Silva, J. (1978). Abnormalities of lymphocytic transformation in women with condylomata acuminata. *Obstetrics & Gynecology*, **51**, 188–92.

Shepherd, P. S., Tran, T. T. T., Rowe, A., Cridland, J. C., Comerford, S. A., Chapman, M. G., and Rayfield, L. S. (1992). T cell responses to the human papillomavirus type 16 E7 protein in mice of different haplotypes. *Journal of General Virology*, **73**, 1269–74.

Stauss, H. J., Davies, D. H., Sadovnikova, E., Horowitz, N., Chain, B. M., and

Sinclair, C. (1992). Induction of cytotoxic T lymphocytes with peptides *in vitro*: Identification of candidate T cell epitopes in human papilloma virus. *Proceedings of the National Academy of Sciences (USA)*, **89**, 7871–5.

Steele, J. C. and Gallimore, P. H. (1990). Humoral anlaysis of human sera to disrupted and non-disrupted epitopes of human papillomavirus type 1. *Virology*, **174**, 388–98.

Strang, G., Hickling, J. K., McIndoe, G. A. J., Howland, K., Wilkinson, D., Ikeda, H. *et al.* (1990). Human T cell responses to human papillomavirus type 16 Ll and E6 synthetic peptides: identification of T cell determinants, HLA-DR restriction and virus type specificity. *Journal of General Virology*, **71**, 423–31.

Suhrbier, A., Scmidt, C., and Fernan, A. (1993). Prediction of an HLA B8-restricted influenza epitope by motif. *Immunology*, **79**, 171–3.

Sumner, J. W., Fekadu, M., Shaddock, J. H., Esposito, J. J., and Bellini, W. J. (1991). Protection of mice with vaccinia virus recombinants that express the rabies nucleoprotein. *Virology*, **183**, 703–10.

Sutton, J., Rowland-Jones, S., Rosenberg, W., Nixon, D., Gotch, F., Gao, X-M., *et al.* (1993). A sequence pattern for peptides presented to cytotoxic T lymphocytes by HLA B8 revealed by analysis of epitopes and eluted peptides. *European Journal of Immunology*, **23**, 447–53.

Syrjänen, K. J. (1989). Histopathology, cytology, immunochemistry and HPV typing techniques. In *Genitoanal papilloma virus infection* (eds. G. von Krogh and E. Rylander) Chapter III, pp. 35–67. Conpharm AB, Karlstad.

Tagami, H., Oku, T., and Iwatsuki, K. (1985). Primary tissue culture of spontaneously regressing flat warts. *In vitro* attack by mononuclear cells against wart-derived epidermal cells. *Cancer*, **55**, 2437–11.

Tarpey, I., Stacey, S., Hickling, J., Birley, H. D. L. Renton, A., McIndoe, A., and Davies, D. H. (1994). Human cytotoxic T lymphocytes stimulated by endogeneously processed human papillomavirus type II E7 recognize a peptide containing a HLA-A2 (A*0201) motif. *Immunology*, **81**, 222–7.

Thivolet, J., Viac, J. and Staquet, M. J. (1982). Cell mediated immunity in wart infection. *International Journal of Dermatology*, **21**, 94.

Tindle, R. W., Fernando, G. J. P., Sterling, J. C., and Frazer, I. H. (1991). A 'public' T-helper epitope of the E7 transforming protein of HPV 16 provides cognate help for several E7 B-cell epitopes from cervical cancer-associated HPV genotypes. *Proceedings of the National Academy of Sciences (USA)*, **88**, 5887–91.

Townsend, A., Rothbard, J., Gotch, F., Bahadur, B., Wraith, D., and McMichael, A. (1986). The epitopes of influenza nucleoprotein recognized by cytotoxic T lymphocytes can be defined with short synthetic peptides. *Cell*, **44**, 959–68.

Townsend, A., Ohlen, C., Bastin J., Ljunggren, H. G., Foster, L., and Karre, K. (1989). Association of class I major histocompatibility heavy and light chains induced by viral peptides. *Nature*, **340**, 443–8.

Van Bleek, G. M. and Nathenson, S. G. (1990). Isolation of an endogenously processed immunodominant viral peptide from the class I H-2K^b molecule. *Nature*, **348**, 213–48.

Viac, J., Chardonnet, Y., Euvard, S., and Schmitt, D. (1992). Epidermotropism of T cells correlates with intracellular adhesion molecule (ICAM 1) expression in human papillomavirus-induced lesions. *Journal of Pathology*, **168**, 301–6.

Zanetti, M., Sercarz, E., and Salk, J. (1987). The immunology of new generation vaccines. *Immunology Today*, **8**, 18–24.

Zhou, J., Sun, X-Y., Stenzel, D. J., and Frazer, I. H. (1991). Expression of vaccinia recombinant HPV 16 L1 and L2 ORF proteins in epithelial cells is sufficient for assembly of HPV virion-like particles. *Virology*, **185**, 251–7.

Zhou, J., Stenzel, D. J., Sun, X-Y., and Frazer, I. H. (1993). Synthesis and assembly of infectious bovine papillomavirus particles *in vitro*. *Journal of General Virology*, **74**, 763–8.

12 Concluding remarks

PETER L. STERN and MARGARET STANLEY

It is clear that HPV infection is a necessary but not sufficient factor in the development of cervical malignancy. The natural history of genital infection with HPV is largely unknown but recent epidemiological studies indicate that infection with HPV is common in adolescents and young adults and is acquired at the onset of sexual activity. The majority of those infected do not develop overt disease and therefore presumably immune defences clear or suppress viral infection. It is not known, in individuals who have been infected, whether the virus persists in a latent state similar to that found with other viruses such as EBV, HSV, and HIV. It is obviously an absolute requirement to determine if latency is a feature of the natural history of HPV infection in the genital tract. Disease is diagnosed by the pathologist by recognition of changes in the individual morphology of cells and changes in the architecture of the tissues but virus may not be present in lesions which histologically are 'warty', or conversely virus can be detected in samples from supposedly normal epithelium. Detection is dependent upon sampling the right tissues from a relevant population and at an appropriate time. The entire genital tract in both men and women may be the reservoir of infection and it may be necessary to sample more extensively (as well as efficiently) in order to properly evaluate the value of HPV DNA detection in the identification of risk groups. An important example of this is the relative position of the squamocolumnar junction in pre-menopausal as opposed to menopausal women. Since this junction is high in the endocervical canal in the latter, effective sampling and detection of virus is therefore more difficult. It is possible that the detection of HPV DNA may be useful in identifying those at risk for progression in premalignant cervical disease but it is obvious that methodological uncertainties remain which need to be resolved. The association and persistence of HPV in high frequency with both pre-malignant and malignant lesions is not in contention and it is this which suggests the possibility of immunological intervention.

The viral mission is to replicate and make infectious particles and transmit them. It does this by hijacking the differentiation process of the normal epithelium, assembling infectious particles only in dead cells ready for exfoliation and transmission. Thus immune intervention to produce virus neutralizing antibodies or cell mediated immunity to clear residually infected cells at this stage in the spectrum of the disease could be effective both as a therapeutic or prophylactic strategy. Many years later the end point of the disease, invasive cervical cancer, is the result of a multistep process which selects transformed immortalized cells which do not terminally differentiate, thus presenting a blind alley for permissive viral growth. However, the continued expression of the viral oncoproteins, E6 and E7, presents opportunities for immunological targeting. At first glance such approaches are very attractive and there is considerable enthusiasm for their implementation *but* . . . .

Examining first the prospects for prophylaxis. HPV is an exclusively intra-epithelial pathogen and we have no idea whether there is a significant viraemia; if there is, when it is, how long it lasts, and whether it is influenced by the endocrine status of the woman and/or the role of other co-factors including viruses such as HSV. What is known of the humoral response in HPV infection suggests that it has little to do with the prevention of infection or the maintenance of latency. This might reflect the fact that while antibodies are made in patients with cervical disease, they are of an inappropriate specificity or are not relevant to mucosal infections. On the bright side, however, in the animal model systems in which virions are produced such as the rabbit and in cattle, immunization with whole virus or capsid proteins is protective. Expression systems are now available which permit the *in vitro* assembly of empty HPV 16 virus-like particles which may express authentic conformational determinants which could evoke a relevant protective serological response; this represents a major development both for good serological and epidemiological studies and in the long term for prophylactic vaccination. There is another problem in that the age at which one is first infected is not established, which poses problems as to when to immunize against capsid antigens. Such immunity may not be very long lived and could have negative influences on immunity to subsequent HPV infections. There is a school of thought which holds that the effective immunity produced by live vaccines is the consequence of a persistent low level of vaccine-derived viral replication. This is apparently not occurring in the natural HPV infection where persistent viral replication is not accompanied by effective immunity. The ultimate prophylactic vaccine would produce both a relevant serological and cell-mediated response. It is not at all clear what the relevant target(s) antigens would be.

To identify potential target antigens one needs to examine the natural history of viral gene expression in relation to epithelial maturation. In the basal layers there is no evidence of viral transcription or proteins but viral proteins must be being expressed since the viral episome is stably maintained in these cells. At present we do not know how to target the virus in the infected stem cell but it is reasonable to assume that the viral early proteins E1,E2, E5, E6, and E7, which are subsequently expressed at high level in the intermediate layers, are viable candidates. Alternative splicing, which is a feature of HPV transcription, may, however, engender stage specific forms of these proteins. This gives an added level of complexity and diversity to the problem of selection of a target antigen. Probably the most abundant viral protein, E4, is only made in large amounts in the most superficial differentiated layers of the epithelium and presents the same problems as the capsid proteins, the cells are dead and eliminating them is not advantageous.

Apparently the differentiation status of the epithelium associated with HPV infection does not preclude CTL recognition of MHC class I restricted antigens. MHC class II expression by the infected keratinocytes, which is frequently found in these cervical lesions, may induce non-responsiveness in CD4 restricted T cells. The dividing line between inducing anergy or effective T cell mediated immunity depends on a combination of antigen presentation with sufficient and appropriate accessory molecules, the concentration of the antigen, the polymorphism of the HLA, and the T cell repertoire. The virus of course has evolved in the face of all these components and succeeds in producing chronic infection. This virus is very frustrating for the immune response because its replication strategy depends upon maintaining the integrity of the infected stem cell. HPV is not cytolytic, the life cycle takes weeks not days to complete, and therefore evasion of immunity is paramount.

If we could identify and validate a prophylactic vaccine, who would we vaccinate? Lets deal with men first. Prevention of infection in men by vaccination of boys before the onset of sexual activity would probably be the most cost-effective approach but of course presupposes that sexual transmission is the only effective route of infection. Therapeutic immunization of women at high risk or with detectable oncogenic HPV infection would be desirable to prevent recurrence from latent reactivation or re-infection. However, there are many viruses and vaccination against the most prevalent types would not provide blanket protection. Nevertheless, if one could significantly reduce the prevalence of cervical disease by vaccination programmes it would have a significant economic and social benefit.

Immunologists always say when faced with no evidence of immunity in cancer that it does not matter because they will be able to induce it. So the question then is can we use the expression of HPV-encoded proteins in cervical cancer to induce immunity against these and thus against the cancer cell even if we are unable to prevent the initial infection? The difficulties in pursuing this approach are very significant given the evidence that many cancers have down-regulated expression of HLA class I alleles and may have other mutations which prevent effective association of the viral peptide and HLA class I peptides. However, CTL directed killing is not the only mechanism for cytotoxicity and strategies which induce more primitive effector responses such as NK cells or macrophages may be relevant in this context. Nonetheless, one is left with the conclusion that to date the virus is proving to be smarter than the biologist.

Index